How the

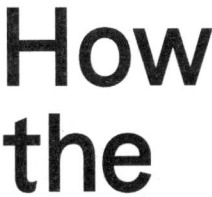

Female
Body
Works

(In all its wild, miraculous glory)

Polly
Vernon

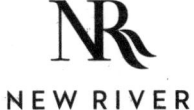

NEW RIVER

Published in 2025 by New River Books
Unit 105, Leroy House, 436 Essex Road, London N1 3QP
www.newriverbooks.co.uk

10 9 8 7 6 5 4 3 2

A CIP catalogue record for this book is available from the British Library.

ISBN: 978-1-915780-07-2

Illustrations by Helena Sutcliffe
Cover design by Emma Ewbank
Interior design by Smith & Gilmour

Printed and Bound in the UK using 100% Renewable Electricity at
CPI Group (UK) Ltd, Croydon, CR0 4YY.

This FSC® label means that materials used for the product have been
responsibly sourced.

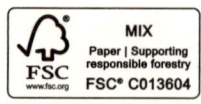

To my goddaughter, Agnes

*(I hereby make good on a promise made on
Christmas Eve, in The Pineapple Pub)*

Contents

INTRODUCTION

How much do you know about the female body? *Your* body? Or, your partner's, your friends', your sister's, your kid's?

Oh, you know the one! It's considered softer, "fairer"; more vulnerable but also, more capable of enduring pain. It bleeds on purpose sometimes, it can get pregnant at others, it's both fetishised and derided (often by the same people, at the same time), and it belongs to 49.7% of the world's population.[1]

Even if two centuries of modern medicine – almost exclusively developed and practised by men – have provided some facts re key organs, what goes where and why (let's not – yet – get into the fact that women's bodies were omitted from US clinical trials from 1977 to 1993, or that, for some years they were routinely considered as smaller, stranger versions of men's bodies)… How much of that knowledge have we absorbed? Fully, or even partially understood?

For example: Do you know what a female sex hormone is? Or *any* hormone for that matter – what they look like, how they operate? What they *want* from us? Are they really our diabolical overlords, capable of manipulating our bodies and our personalities on an unknowable whim? Or are they on-side? Supportive? Friendly, even?

---

1 Population, female (% of total population), World Bank, 2024 – https://data.worldbank.org/indicator/SP.POP.TOTL.FE.ZS

And what's a brain? Because, while my knowledge of that especially essential organ settles somewhere between it's-the-bit-where-I-get-my-thinking-done, and, it's-bulbous-and-veiny-and-divided-into-two, I also appreciate, this isn't really adequate. What's it *made* of? Is a female brain distinct from a male brain?

Did you know women are twice as likely to be diagnosed with depression and Alzheimer's?

Oh, and: might we talk about boobs? What they're made of, how much they cost a woman over the course of her life, and how on earth they produce milk?

And the vagina, (which, by the way, is not the same thing as the vulva – did you know that? Because I didn't!)

And then, there's the pelvic floor and the fallopian tubes and – it's a wild geographical segue I appreciate, *but*: wouldn't it be good to know why woman footballers are so much more likely than men to tear their ACLs? That's the anterior cruciate ligament, which resides in the knee. And what does that mean if you're not a woman footballer, just, y'know, a *woman*?

And I've always wondered what a period *really* is. Sure: I know about the pain, the feeling like you're being kicked repeatedly in the ovaries from the inside, and I know about the blood and (on occasion) the abject relief you're not pregnant, and (on others) the terrible sadness because you're not pregnant, but, what I'm asking here, honestly, is: *how does it happen?* What's the *mechanism*?

And why do you feel like seven shades of worthless crap just before them, then, like several gazillion dollars of competent, sexy, gregarious wonder, just a little later? And why do they stop, not just in menopause?

And what is menopause? Is it puberty in reverse? An initially slow, but then increasingly speedy luge run towards pointlessness, social invisibility, crumbly bones, a mushed-up brain, fury, flushes, divorce and death?

Or is it actually not that at all? Because, you know, women have been known to win Nobel Prizes after the menopause.

Back to puberty though, because it impacts girls differently. Some say it's worse, some say it's better. There's certainly an idea that girls mature faster than boys… But maybe that's just something we say, to keep them in line. And why does childbirth hurt so damn much? What's the logic in that? Wouldn't it be more sensible – for the continuation of the species and so forth – for childbirth to be, I dunno: *fun*? How is breast milk made? Does it really vary in formulation according to what your baby needs, from feed to feed? How much extra does it cost a person to have a pair of breasts over the course of a lifetime, in terms of bras, milk pumps and back pain, possible cancer treatment, and so on? It's gotta be a few grand, right? In which case: should we have tax breaks on boobs?

And another hot topic: infertility. Is it more common now, or are we just more aware of it, partly thanks to the lucrative industry built around fixing it? Why is everyone freezing their eggs? Should you freeze yours? What's that like? Does it hurt?

How does the pill work? No, really? And is it actually bad for you? Why is TikTok alight with claims like: "Birth control is this generation's smoking"; is it really associated with an increased risk of suicide? Or is it the most freeing, empowering thing to happen to women since we won the right to vote? As one doctor put it to a friend of mine who'd asked if she should stop taking the pill and embrace a more "natural" life:

"Natural? You wanna know what natural is, for a woman? It's getting pregnant and giving birth, over and over and over again, from puberty to menopause, at which point you'll die of exhaustion – assuming you haven't already died in childbirth, of course. That's what 'natural' is."

I didn't know. Didn't know any of it. For years, I'd driven my body around like it was a car – and I had zero interest in the manual. Then, one day last year, I found myself in the haematology department of my local hospital – The Whittington, North London – waiting for a blood test. I was due to start taking a drug to cure a dose of toenail fungus, sexy I know; this drug was hardcore enough that my liver function needed to be assessed in advance. There were, I dunno, 40-ish people in the waiting room with me, all ages, all ethnicities, all shapes and sizes and clothing choices and so on and so forth, but… just the one gender. We were all female. Every last one of us.

"What's this about?" I wondered.

Later that day: I loitered on a tube platform, waiting for my train, half-heartedly reading the billboard adverts covering the walls. I suddenly realised that one in three of them – maybe more – were offering private diagnostic tests. There was everything, from fertility tests, menopause-related hormone tests and immune system tests to thyroid function. There were "peace of mind full body health checks", there was a sort of upright cubicle device, a bit like an airport security system, offering non-specific full body scans.

All these tests! All several hundred quid a pop, by my guess, but here's my point: almost all of them were very obviously aimed at women. Tests designed to check every aspect of us, to pinpoint potential failings and deficiencies, and name and quantify future risks we hadn't even considered, yet.

"Freeze now. Live today. Try later," ran one, an ad for egg freezing services.

"One in two women aged over 50 will break a bone due to poor bone health," read yet another.

Blimey, I thought.

Suddenly, it was like I'd tuned into a radio station that was back-to-back chat about women's bodies. "There's more research into male patent baldness, than there is into all aspects of women's health combined," a health-fixated feminist mate tells me. "Also: guess what the second biggest demographic for STIs – sexually transmitted infections – after teenage girls and young 20-something women is? It's women in their 40s and 50s!"

"Older! They're turning up with chlamydia in their 50s and 60s," says Dr Kate Jolowicz, my local GP, a rock star of a practitioner (genuinely, people queue to see her). "Did you also know that more sanitary pads are sold to women with incontinence because of pelvic floor issues, than for their periods?"

I did not.

A heavily pregnant friend tells me she had to have two counselling sessions before medics would consider giving her the elective caesarean she had, following careful consideration, decided she wanted. One midwife told her that she wouldn't bond with her baby as well, if it were born through caesarean birth.

Could that be true?

My physio mate, Wendy, says they used to give teenage girls

oestrogen if they thought they were growing too tall ("In the 70s! Not that long ago!"). The psychologist in my local coffee shop tells me it's "Bullsh*t that women have a higher pain threshold. We just put up with more pain."

"Are we really twice as depressed as men?" I ask her. "Or are women just more likely to seek help?"

"Isn't that the million-dollar question," she says.

"Did you know there's evidence hormone replacement therapy (HRT) protects against dementia, heart disease, strokes *and* osteoporosis?" Dr Jolowicz tells me.

"But isn't it a bit dangerous?" I say. "I thought it was dangerous. Why do I think it's dangerous?"

"There was a discredited study in the 90s. Look it up."

"Yeah, but HRT's also been massively over-prescribed lately," says my frenemy the wellness influencer. "It's a scandal. Did you know that male babies only become male at six to seven weeks gestation? And that girl babies are usually stronger than boy babies in the early stages of development, with a lower chance of complications?"

And so on and so forth and so damn overwhelming and confusing and contradictory that I start feeling like I need some definitive answers. Desperately.

I'm a journalist, an interviewer by trade. I've interviewed everyone from Donald Trump to Gwyneth Paltrow. Interviewing is something I love doing; lifting the bonnet on someone else's mind, having a good old rummage, seeing who they are and what they know. It's one of the few things I'm qualified to do, too.

So – I started thinking – what if I were to apply my interview techniques to a load of experts in women's bodies? Neuroscientists, academics, medical specialists, midwives, gynaes, psychologists and physios? What if I were to layer up different perspectives on the same topics, and compare and contrast ideas and experiences? What if I were to collate... Not just the textbook knowledge, but also the evolving theses, observations and personal experiences of a bunch of people who have dedicated their professional lives to women's bodies?

What if I were to ask all the people who actually know – the people at the (sometimes, literally) beating heart of it – *How the Female Body Works*?

What if we could chart the scope, track how it changes across a lifetime? From puberty – the point where I guess we could say it first becomes functionally female – through the childbearing years and on. Through the real meaning and impact of the menstrual cycle, to fertility, and the issues it brings, then: pregnancy and childbirth, perimenopause, menopause, and older age. What if, together, we were to unpack the messiness and beauty, the complexities and mysteries, and gain a better understanding of what happens when an aspect of it doesn't work, along with the magnificence and power of when it *does*? How it waxes and wanes, shifts and transforms, from day to day to week to month to year to decade? What if we dug deep – my experts and I – into the wild and miraculous glory of female bodies, of *our* bodies?

Might that be useful? Fascinating? Challenging, surprising, funny, infuriating, revelatory, reassuring?

Might that be... *amazing*?

A NOTE ABOUT MY EXPERTS

I did not intend for this to be a political book. I really didn't. I just wanted it to be useful, and I thought factual beats political in that respect, every time. But. It turns out it's fantastically difficult to contemplate women's bodies, and by extension, women's health, without also getting political. Politics is just... *there*. For example: from the very beginning of medicine, women were presumed physically inferior to men – Aristotle called us the "mutilated male". This jumping off point led, inevitably, to the proliferation in the 18th and 19th centuries of ideas like "hysteria" – the belief that everything from epilepsy to what we now call borderline personality disorder could be blamed on the womb. Add to that a vague, persistent ickiness around female hormones, and a general lack of desire to engage with them in any meaningful way. Doctors and researchers were historically male, which meant the female experience was inevitably and completely underrepresented; most of the cells – animal as well as human – studied by medical science were also male. In 1977, the American Food and Drug Administration formally excluded all women of childbearing age from all drug trials following a series of drug-related disasters, most strikingly, the thalidomide tragedy.[2] This led to vast shortages of data on how drugs impacted women, something which only began to be corrected in 1993, when the inclusion of women and minority groups in trials was legally mandated in the US. "We literally know less about every aspect of female biology compared to male biology," Dr Janine Austin Clayton, associate director for

---

2 Thalidomide-induced teratogenesis: history and mechanisms, *Birth Defects Res C Embryo Today*, 2015 – https://www.ncbi.nlm.nih.gov/pmc/articles/PMC4737249

women's health research at the US National Institutes of Health, told the New York Times in 2014.

If things are changing, and some of them are, they're changing slowly. And some of them are not changing. Some are getting worse: according to a 2023 study by the painkiller brand Nurofen, the gender gap on pain – the ways in which, and extent to which, women suffer more pain than men – is getting wider. All of this has led to a lot of understandable fury about how overlooked women and our bodies have been. How disregarded, how – at best – reduced to our biological function, and ignored beyond that. How let down. How… allowed to die.

But I'll tell you something about the experts I interviewed for this book: they convinced me that this absence of care, of concern, of research into female bodies, this scientific wariness of them – is categorically not the whole story. Every last one of my experts showed themselves to be gentle but ferocious warriors in the war against what has recently been named "medical misogyny" – an umbrella term for the systemic gaps in knowledge, interest and treatment when it comes to women's bodies.

In their every word, their every sigh and pause, in how passionate they became, how excited and (sometimes) furious, and in all the extreme patience they showed me (as I tried my very hardest to keep up), my experts showed me nothing but the purest respect for female bodies. Passion. Reverence. Delight. Extraordinary care. A deep desire to help, to heal. I was left with the same sense, after speaking to each and every one of them: love. True *love* for women's bodies.

It made me feel very hopeful.

CHAPTER ONE

WHAT ACTUALLY ARE HORMONES?

Where else could I start my exploration of female bodies but with hormones?

What's that, you say? Breasts? Yeah, maybe. They too are routinely used as a shorthand for the condition of femaleness – ah, but, you know what? No. Because it takes hormones to make breasts in the first place; without hormones, there just is no female body.

So: what are they? I hear them invoked over and over as the root cause of everything – from low mood to poor sleep, from spots to a random itch, an intense headache, how alluring we appear to the world, or how reclusive we feel from it. Our worst tempers, our weirdest outbursts, our joys and sorrows (the full range of our emotional responses, actually), our excessive sweating, sudden changes in smell, pregnancy, infertility, periods – and the end of them – hormones are the cause of it all.

They're like a bunch of unknowable Greek Gods, buffeting our bodies and emotions around, according to their will.

But where do they come from? And how do they work? Are we born with them? Like, with a store of them? Do they lurk in our children's bodies, waiting for puberty to wake them up? Can you see them under a microscope? In which case – do different hormones look different? Can we *smell* them?

Above all else, I think: how responsible are they for our characters? Our personalities? Do hormones make us who we are? More, or less, emotional? Or anxious? Or angry?

This question starts to overwhelm me, and I end up wondering: am I me? Or am I my hormones?

* * *

I first hear of Dr Nicky Keay after finding a paper she wrote on stress fractures in female athletes and ballet dancers whose periods had stopped because of undereating and overtraining. I google Keay and discover she's a trained doctor, a lecturer in hormones at University College London and an advisor to dance companies, working closely with dancers to study their menstrual cycles and the impact they have on their performance. She's also the author of *Hormones, Health and Human Potential*, published in 2022, and *Myths of Menopause*, 2024.

I email her and ask if she'd meet. She says yes – "Always happy to talk hormones!" – and invites me to her home in south London for coffee. She takes me on a tour of the mini dance studio she has set up in a back room, complete with a mirror, practice barre and a section of hardwood floor taken from English National Ballet offcuts ("my husband thought it was a daft idea, then Covid hit, ha!").

I ask her what a hormone is.

"It's a molecule that travels around in your bloodstream. The word comes from ancient Greek; it means: 'setting in motion'. What's it setting in motion? Your DNA. Your blueprint for life."

DNA, or deoxyribonucleic acid, holds the instructions for

building and running our bodies. It is made of two linked strands that wind around each other to resemble a twisted ladder – a shape known as a double helix. Hormones tell our cells which part of the DNA to read and how to put those instructions to work.

So, I ask, is our DNA loitering in our cells, waiting for our hormones to boot them into action?

"Exactly!"

What's a hormone made of?

"On an atomic level? Carbon, hydrogen and oxygen with some 'optional' other elements." Dr Keay goes on to explain that there are two types of hormone: protein and steroid. Protein hormones are made from amino acids, while steroid hormones, aka the sex hormones – oestrogen, progesterone and testosterone – are made from cholesterol. Some hormones exist in our bodies from when we are in the womb, and others, including the sex hormones, the ones that make our bodies male or female, kick in later, in puberty.

"A hormone," says Dr Charlotte Gribbin, a doctor of aesthetics and regenerative medicine – Botox, filler, and so forth – whose work by definition brings her into contact with many women in their 40s and 50s, so is often underpinned by whatever the hell is happening with their hormones, "is produced by a gland. It causes an effect somewhere."

You could think of hormones as a messaging system, I learn. They're like chemical telegrams, which zip from the gland to an organ, prompting it to perform a function.

It triggers the process of you growing a pair of boobs or starting your period, or prepares your body for pregnancy.

Some hormones work slowly, methodically, and according to a schedule. They send you to sleep at night (melatonin) and wake you in the morning (cortisol). Others are more instant and are inspired by a change in your environment. Adrenaline would be an example.

"Adrenaline comes from the adrenal glands," Dr Gribbin says. These are small, triangular-shaped glands that sit on top of the kidneys and produce various hormones that regulate your metabolism, immune system, blood pressure and, in the case of adrenaline, your response to alarming situations. Adrenaline, like melatonin and cortisol, are also examples of hormones that act on your body through childhood.

The human body produces a lot of hormones, over 50 by current medical reckoning. They exist within the endocrine system, communicating with each other and moderating the quantities released at any one time in accordance with each other.

Dr Gribbin explains that hormones are different from neurotransmitters – like dopamine and serotonin. Neurotransmitters are chemicals released between nerve cells in the brain. "Hormones talk to each other. Like, if you have too much dopamine, it's not going to go back to your brain and say: 'I have enough now, don't produce anymore'. Whereas, if you have enough oestrogen, that's going to feedback and say: 'Stop now. I need you to cool it for a while.'" Whatever else it does, your body is constantly working away in the background, beyond your consciousness, ensuring you're neither too hot, nor too cold, too thirsty, or overhydrated. Hormones are part of that system.

That's so clever.

"Oh, hormones are very clever," says Dr Keay. "There are whole families of them! An orchestra is how I describe them, imagine the strings, the woodwind – they're all in there, in their little group. Overall, they make a whole symphony." (Dr Keay – music lover, ballet devotee – generally thinks of hormones in terms of music and dance.)

Men and women share pretty much all of them; they just produce them in greater or lesser quantities.

Hormonal fluctuations are thought to be behind sleep troubles in women, which may explain why men tend to experience less insomnia. Interestingly, some studies suggest that women generally sleep better than men[1] – though they also need more sleep overall.

Men and women both produce adrenaline, as discussed; and cortisol, another stress hormone, which also comes from the adrenal glands – although some studies have shown that men have a higher baseline level of this. Cortisol is, as we've seen, responsible for waking you in the morning.

And incidentally, Dr Gribbin tells me the most common time of the day for both men and women to have a heart attack is between seven and eight in the morning, when cortisol peaks.

Cortisol controls your body's response to a stressful situation by increasing the sugar (glucose) in your bloodstream, on the assumption it will prove useful in a fight-or-flight situation, powering muscles to punch and/or run, then managing their subsequent

---

1 Women sleep objectively better than men and the sleep of young women is more resilient to external stressors, *J Sleep Res*, 2009 – https://pmc.ncbi.nlm.nih.gov/articles/PMC3594776/

repair. This is fabulous if you *are* in a fight-or-flight situation, but not so great if you're not – if your stress is related to, say, a relentless onslaught of emails, road rage or undernourishing your body for an extended period of time in a misguided, desperate attempt to lose weight, because there's a party or you want to have a beach body. And of course you know *intellectually* your self-worth should not be even fleetingly associated with your dress size, but you've got millennia of cultural expectation to overturn before you feel that instinctually – and a crash diet will be quicker.

And yet, according to Dr Keay, cortisol is the reason extreme diets don't work. If you allow your calorific intake to drop suddenly and sharply with one of those diets, your body will respond by increasing cortisol, which – oh, irony! – encourages it to store fat in the assumption that you're in some sort of emergency situation. A famine, perhaps. Cortisol-related weight gain tends to result in fat lodged around your abdomen, your stomach, waist, lower back – and in you weighing more than you did, before you started the crash diet.

Oxytocin is the cuddler's hormone, the warm and fuzzy hormone, the bonder, the lover; it's released into the bloodstream by the hypothalamus – a big daddy of a gland, a hormonal overlord situated in your brain – in response to anything from breastfeeding your newborn baby, to stroking a dog, to having an orgasm. Oxytocin literally makes you warm, too – it's involved in the thermoregulation of your body, which is, presumably, why we associate it with emotional warmth.

Insulin is produced in the pancreas – the six-inch section of your digestive system located in your upper abdomen, behind the stomach – and regulates how effectively your cells use the glucose in your bloodstream, which is why a lack of it, or an inability to use it well, is associated with type 1 and type 2 diabetes.

T3 (triiodothyronine) and T4 (thyroxine) are the main thyroid hormones, produced by – you guessed it – the thyroid, the butterfly-shaped gland that lies against and wraps around your windpipe. T3 and T4 are responsible for regulating your metabolism, your digestive processes, your hunger and your related energy levels.

Melatonin, like cortisol, is essential to your cycle of sleeping and waking, also known as your circadian rhythm. Melatonin originates in the pineal gland, which is located deep in the brain. It's activated at night by a depletion in sunlight, which is why you get sleepy after dark, and it's at its lowest levels in your body in the morning, when cortisol is at its highest. NB: blue light emitted by laptops, smartphones and tablets had, until recently, been widely assumed to suppress melatonin, and in turn, disrupt sleep. However, a new review published in 2024 in the journal *Sleep Medicine Reviews*,[2] and drawing on 11 studies, concluded this is probably not the case; it's more likely that being deeply absorbed by whatever it is we're scrolling through, and thus neglecting to focus on falling asleep, is what's actually causing the disruption.

Then come the sex hormones, the steroid hormones – oestrogen, progesterone and testosterone – which don't bother your body much until it hits puberty. We're getting to them, cool your boots.

Can we smell hormones? Adrenaline: in a way, yes. There are

---

2 A bidirectional model of sleep and technology use, *Sleep Medicine Reviews*, 2024 – https://doi.org/10.1016/j.smrv.2024.101933

two distinct varieties of sweat gland: eccrine, which occur all over your body and secrete the looser, more watery, less pungent kind of sweat designed to cool you down after physical exertion, and apocrine, which tends to limit itself to the armpit area. The apocrine sweat gland is activated uniquely by psychological stress, and the sweat it produces is much denser and more viscous. Apocrine gland sweat also smells stronger, and it has a sulphurous undertone; there's some scientific conjecture that it evolved as a way of communicating potential danger across tribes. Regardless, it certainly accounts for the rank aroma emitted by the entire planeload of holidaymakers that time I arrived in Malaga airport following three failed landing attempts (crosswinds on the runway, loves!), whose armpits betrayed any and all communal attempts to keep a lid on abject panic.

As for *arôme de* oestrogen, according to an (admittedly small) 2019 study from the University of Zurich, in which men were asked to rate 28 women of reproductive age in order of the attractiveness of their smell: yes, we can. All the study subjects chose women who, previous tests indicated, possessed the highest levels of oestrogen. Another study by researchers at Yale University, published in 2020,[3] designed to challenge the prevailing idea that a woman's facial symmetry alters to become more attractive during the peak of her menstrual cycle, when her hormone levels are at their highest, concluded it was more likely that women simply smell different when they are most fertile.

Can we see hormones under a microscope? Nope. You can see the red blood cells they zip about in, but hormones themselves

---

3 Stability of women's facial shape throughout the menstrual cycle, *Proc Biol Sci.*, 2020 – https://pubmed.ncbi.nlm.nih.gov/32259474/

are not visible. Scientists have, however, mapped them out as chemical structures.

"Let me show you a hormone spinning round," says Dr Keay. She produces a laptop. A vertical structure of interlocking hexagons with outstretched arms and tipped with red dots dances around in front of us. It's oestradiol, one of oestrogen's three forms; it's most potent incarnation.

"It's a beautiful molecule," Dr Keay sighs. "It's my favourite."

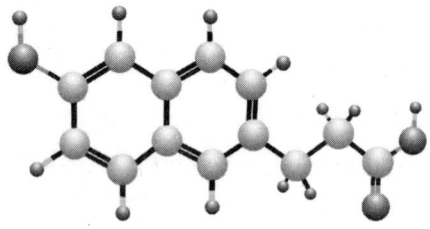

It seems like the right moment to ask the question that's been obsessing me more and more lately, so I grab it:

How much of our personality do hormones account for? Like: how much of us is *us*, and how much is our hormones? Are "female" hormones responsible for those things so routinely described as feminine traits? Does more oestrogen make us more caring, for example, more loving, more desiring of closeness and bonding? More inclined to look after others? Or is that about us having less testosterone? Or is it about oxytocin, the cuddly, orgasmy hormone, present in higher levels in women than men?[4]

Does the particular female hormone mix really make us moodier,

4 Sex-related differences in plasma oxytocin levels in humans, *Clin Pract Epidemiol Ment Health*, 2019 – https://doi.org/10.2174/1745017901915010058

less reliable, less capable, as is (still) widely presumed? Does it drive our behaviours, our life choices? Make us end relationships we should stay in, storm out of jobs we should also stay in? Or is that sexist bullsh*t and/or social conditioning? And how much of it is about the individual; her specific hormonal mix, her sensitivity to it?

And if not, are women as guilty for perpetuating these ideas as men? For loudly decrying our failings, our inadequacies, our foul tempers, our sadnesses et cetera, blaming it all on our hormones and thus, often, undermining our own position, when bulldozing on through, exuding confidence and competence while appreciating that literally everyone messes up from time to time, while never once mentioning our hormones, might serve us far better?

Above all: *where do our hormones end, and where does our actual, essential us-ness begin?*

"Well, isn't that the question?" Nicky Keay says.

We will be returning to this in the next chapter. Believe.

WHAT I KNOW NOW

- Hormones are chemical messengers, carrying instructions from one part of the body to another.

- There are over 50 hormones in the body.

- Our capacity to produce them is with us in the womb. Through childhood, we're subject to a lot of them, such as melatonin and cortisol, which helps to synchronise our circadian rhythms. Sex hormones begin to impact us in puberty.

- Men and women have the same hormones, just in greater

or lesser quantities.

- We can't see them – but we *can* smell some of them.

- How deeply they define our character and direct our choices is a vast question – one to which I shall be returning, over and over.

CHAPTER TWO

PUBERTY

Right now, I feel like Keanu Reeves in the 90s sci-fi classic *The Matrix*, after he has files of new knowledge downloaded directly into his brain, and he looks up at Morpheus (Laurence Fishburne) and says: "I know Kung-fu."

Only in my case it's: "I know hormones." Sort of, anyway.

What I need to learn about now is sex hormones specifically. The ones that shape women in so many senses, not least how our bodies look and behave.

My vague understanding of them is that they've got something to do with puberty.

What I am about to learn is that sex hormones *are* puberty. And puberty is sex hormones.

★ ★ ★

I meet Dr Charlotte Gribbin at her private clinic, a cool suite of rooms in central London. Dr Gribbin – demonstrative, Irish, instantly likeable – tells me about the earliest stages of her career. She studied medicine, specialising in cardiology, in the mid-90s – around the time medical science first started noticing that women experience heart attacks in different ways from men. Most notably, their symptoms are different. According to Dr Gribbin, "myocardial infarction – the clinical term for a heart attack – was always defined in textbooks by the way it occurs in a man. So I [as a student] was learning typically male symptoms: crushing chest pain, radiating down the left arm, breathlessness, sweatiness… There was a list. *That* person walks into A&E? You're popping an ECG on them! Women, as in every aspect of medicine, present more quietly. A myocardial infarction in a woman is less dramatic. Less loud."

Why?

"Because they make less of a fuss."

Their bodies – our bodies, *women's* bodies – make less fuss? Even when we're having a heart attack and quite possibly dying?

"Yes. Literally. Physically. Audibly. Less fuss."

I think this is incredibly important, so bear with me while I veer completely off topic to explain how a woman might experience a heart attack – a myocardial infarction – and how that might differ from a man's experience of it.

During a heart attack, women are more likely than men to experience nausea and sweating; pain or pressure in parts of the body other than the chest (NB: we might not experience any chest pain at all), for example, in the upper abdomen, jaw, neck or upper back; shortness of breath, fainting, indigestion and extreme fatigue. You should, of course, seek immediate medical assistance if you experience any of these symptoms because *you may be having a heart attack.*

And now – puberty, which I understand as the release into the body of the sex hormones oestrogen and progesterone in the case of girls, which, over the course of a few years, change a child's body into that of an adult, i.e. one physically (though probably not yet emotionally, never mind, financially) capable of sexual reproduction. This feels like a hot mess of psychological and physical turmoil – a tsunami of doubt and boobs, obsession, confusion, perpetual gnawing, soul-seeping FOMO, alienation, nameless, shapeless all-encompassing shame, spots, but also the sparkly, glimmerous foreshadowing of the wondrous, endless possibilities of the life to come – all crashing down over your head and your rapidly changing body over and over again, for four or five years straight. It is exhausting and wildly confusing, though you can take the edge off it, in my experience, by drawing on the Bounty of Superdrug (my gratitude to Clearasil – go-to OTC spot treatment of the 80s – endures).

"Puberty, in fact, is organised, and it is predictable," Dr Gribbin tells me. "It follows a pre-programmed path. An order."

Didn't bloody feel like it, I say.

"Ha!"

She produces a neat, stapled print-out of an academic paper entitled "Physiology, Puberty", published by researchers Logen Breehl and Omar Caban, most recently updated in April 2022. She passes it over.

"It's the best I've read."

"Puberty," the paper begins, "is the process of physical maturation where an adolescent reaches sexual maturity and becomes capable of reproduction. On average, puberty typically begins between eight and 13 in females and nine and 14 in males. Puberty is associated with emotional and hormonal changes, as well as physical changes such as breast development in females (thelarche), pubic hair development (pubarche) … and the onset of menstruation (menarche). Puberty proceeds through five stages, termed Tanner stages, ranging from prepubertal, to full maturity."

The Tanner stages – a scale for measuring the physical development of children as they transition through adolescence into adulthood – were developed by British paediatrician James Tanner in 1969, after he'd spent some 20 years studying the physical changes in girls in puberty. They're still considered the gold standard on pubertal development, widely invoked in research and clinical practice.

TANNER STAGE	DEVELOPMENTS
STAGE 1: *Prepubescent*	• No pubic hair • No breast development
STAGE 2: *Pubarche* *Thelarche*	• Fine pubic hair appears • Breast buds form
STAGE 3: *Pubescent*	• Pubic hair darkens and curls • Breasts enlarge • Growth spurt begins
STAGE 4: *Menarche*	• Adult pubic hair • Areola enlargement • Menarche may occur
STAGE 5: *Postpubescent*	• Pubic hair reaches inner thighs • Fully developed breasts • Adult body shape established

In terms of what happens, when: Stage 2, thelarche, the very beginnings of breasts – the dawn of boobs – tends to kick in between the ages of eight and 11; Stage 4 (menarche) takes effect up to three years later; although environment, nutrition and genetics can impact the timings and progression significantly, sometimes still within the range of healthy and expected, though sometimes not. Dr Philippa Kaye, the GP with whom I speak about the development, function and politics of boobs (Chapter 5), suggests in her book *Breasts, An Owner's Guide* that "if you have not started to develop breasts by age 13… or you develop breasts, but have not started your periods by 15, then please see your doctor."

Puberty starts when the sex hormones – in girls, oestrogen and progesterone, though we do also have some male sex hormone testosterone – are released into our systems.

How?

"GnRH," says Dr Gribbin. "It's the master switch."

Cool, cool. Yeah, no, *what*?

"Gonadotropin-releasing hormone. The clue's in the name. 'Gonad', the gland which produces sex hormones, male and female; 'tropin', that means 'towards' or 'stimulating', and 'hormone'… So, it's a hormone that stimulates the gonad."

In women, the gonads are the ovaries, while in men, they are the testes. These glands control big puberty milestones such as thelarche (the onset of breast development, Tanner Stage 2); pubarche (the appearance of pubic hair, Tanner Stage 2, followed by thickening and coarsening in Stage 3); and menarche (the onset of menstruation, which usually occurs around Tanner Stage 4).

GnRH is released by the hypothalamus, deep in the brain, which in turn controls the function of the pituitary, a pea-sized gland positioned at the base of your brain and in line with your nose. The hypothalamus and the pituitary, which are connected by a cord composed of blood vessels and nerves, work together to keep your body in a state of homeostasis, or self-regulation, to achieve the kind of balance that maximises your chances of survival. Homeostasis is the function, for example, which enables our bodies to maintain a temperature of around 37°C, because this, among many other things, makes it harder for fungal species to thrive within us. Fungi like it cold. (Anyone who has watched the post-apocalyptic wonder TV drama *The Last of Us*, or played the video game on which it was based, will be *so* glad to know this; I know I was.) The hypothalamus and the pituitary are also the ultimate bosses of the endocrine system, overseeing and regulating the production of all hormones in your body.

Around a year before the release of GnRH, i.e. a year before puberty begins, your body will experience adrenarche. As Dr Gribbin explains, this is when "your adrenal gland kicks in, sending a signal to the body: get ready, because once I've done my thing – 'adrenarche', where 'arche' means 'a transitional phase' – GnRH will hit." Adrenarche is a stirring, an awakening, a readying, of the adrenal gland for the onset of puberty.

As puberty begins, GnRH orders the pituitary gland to produce FSH – follicle-stimulating hormone – and LH – luteinising hormone. (I know, I know, I'm bombarding you with acronyms, stick with me, I swear they'll become as familiar as "LOL" or "BRB" or "OOO" in time.) FSH is the hormone responsible for kickstarting egg development. One of the few facts I knew about the female body before I launched myself on this enterprise – I heard it once, and was so creeped out that it stayed with me – is that baby girls are born with all their eggs, the unfertilised bases of pregnancy for an entire lifetime, already in them. These eggs are made while she's still in the womb, which means the egg you came from was actually formed in your maternal grandmother's womb. This is why we can see the impact of things like alcohol consumption across generations.

Women are born with between one and four million eggs, but that number declines over the years. Lots of eggs die off naturally in childhood: 10,000-ish a month, all of which are absorbed back into the body.

By puberty, you're left with somewhere between 40,000 and one million eggs, one (maybe two) a month of which will leave your body when you have your period, while the rest keep right on dying and being absorbed. By the age of 25, we have a paltry 300,000 left, after which, the decline in their numbers gets steeper and steeper until menopause, when they're all gone.

Where was I?

Oh yes.

So GnRH sends its homing pigeons FSH and LH whizzing through the bloodstream, straight to their predetermined destination, the ovaries and the uterus (or womb), where they fly slap bang into the receptors designed to recognise and respond to them. Your ovaries – home to the follicles, the small, fluid-filled sacs that store all those eggs you were born with – receive FSH and LH as an instruction to start producing the sex hormone oestrogen, while the uterus receives them as an instruction to start producing progesterone, and: huzzah! Puberty is launched, like a proud ship, onto the waves of sexual maturity.

But hang on a sweet sec: we need to contemplate female sex hormones more fully. Oestrogen – estrogen, if you're American – is a hormone whose Wikipedia page reads: "Estrogen or oestrogen is a category of sex hormone responsible for the development and regulation of the female reproductive system and secondary sex characteristics." (The female reproductive system, our vagina, uterus, fallopian tubes, clitoris, cervix, along with our capacity to give birth and menstruate are our "primary sex characteristics", while our boobs, broadened hips and underarm and pubic hair are our "secondary sex characteristics").

But this, honestly, is to undersell it tragically.

For oestrogen is the goddess hormone.

Maisie Hill, menstrual health expert, period coach, podcaster and author of *Period Power* (2019), calls it "the Beyoncé of hormones… Confident, alluring, sexy and ready to conquer the world. Oestrogen wants us out there in the world, on the look-out for someone to mate with." Dr Nicky Keay calls it her "favourite". Fertility site Hertility.com calls it "the matriarch". You might *also* consider it "the hussy hormone": a thrilling 2009 study lead by Dr Kristina Durante at the University of Texas claims that, not only do we feel more attractive with more oestrogen in our system [more on this in Chapter 3, The Menstrual Cycle], we're more likely to have illicit affairs on account of it. "Women with higher oestradiol [the most potent variety of oestrogen] reported a greater likelihood of flirting, kissing and having a serious affair with someone other than their primary partner and were marginally more likely to date another man… Our results are consistent with the possibility that highly fertile women [i.e. women with more oestrogen] are not easily satisfied by their long-term partners and are especially motivated to become acquainted with other, presumably more desirable, men."

Oh, but oestrogen is potent! Also, multi-functional. Oestrogen's functions include, but are not limited to: increasing the production of neurotransmitters serotonin and dopamine, which regulate our mood; protecting our nerves and our brains from damage; stimulating the production of hyaluronic acid, collagen and elastin, proteins which, anyone familiar with the Bounty of Superdrug (or Selfridges beauty hall, or cultbeauty. com or really the label on the back of any half-decent moisturiser) will know, makes your skin elastic, bouncy, dewy, pretty. Oestrogen is also responsible for promoting bone mass, thereby protecting them from breaks and fractures; regulating cholesterol, thereby protecting us from heart disease; maintaining the health and thickness of vaginal tissue, keeping it lubricated, stopping it from getting dry. And all this is merely a side hustle to creating and regulating the menstrual cycle and overseeing and supporting pregnancies: specifically, the development of a baby's organs and the function of the placenta. Our bodies, by the way, are flooded with oestrogen when we're pregnant. As neuroscientist Dr Sarah McKay tells me: "If you have a pregnancy, you'll get a thousand times more oestrogen than you'll receive *in the entire rest of your life.*"

You might see oestrogen as a fearless, fun-loving, thrill-seeking dynamo. Progesterone, meanwhile, is like oestrogen's risk-averse, strict, judgemental best friend.

Or perhaps, oestrogen's manager? Progesterone is subtler, quieter – but in a powerful way, not a shy way – and it's mysterious. "We don't really understand as much about it," Dr McKay says. Oestrogen would be nothing without progesterone. They're an interdependent double act, more on this to come (see Chapter 3, The Menstrual Cycle).

So. Puberty. It is now, Dr Gribbin explains, that oestrogen starts to act on the ovaries for the very first time, while progesterone starts to act on the uterus. This means that the ovaries will start to stimulate one or two of those eggs into a state of maturity, ready for release into the fallopian tubes, while the endometrial lining on the uterus will thicken. The uterus itself will enlarge. This is because production of your growth hormone increases in puberty – doubles, in fact[5] – which means your body extends: your bones literally lengthen.

One of the powerful impacts growth hormones have on the female body is that it broadens our hips, which in turn, results in a greater Q-angle. The Q-angle, or quadriceps angle, is an imaginary line used as a reference point by medics. It runs between the pelvis through the quadriceps – the big muscles in the front of your thighs – and down into the patella tendons in the knee. The Q-angle in women is around 13–18 degrees, as compared to around 12–15 degrees in men. While the broader hips associated with the greater Q-angle are useful in terms of giving birth, they're less so when it comes to physical sport, where they seem to increase the likelihood of injuries. More on this, soon.

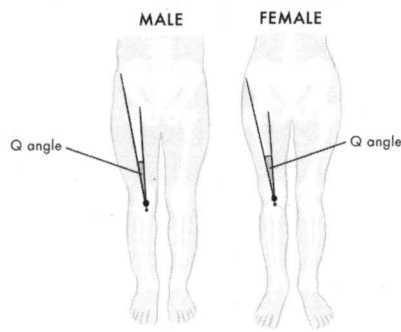

Then comes some visible evidence of puberty: thelarche, which is when oestrogen kickstarts the growing of breasts.

About six months after thelarche, comes pubarche, the development of pubic hair (which is initially sparse and fine,

5 Dose effects of growth hormone during puberty, *Horm Res.*, 2003 – https://pubmed.ncbi.nlm.nih.gov/12955018/

according to Tanner Stage 2). This occurs in response to the production of adrenal androgens, male sex hormones secreted by the adrenal glands in both men and women. "Sex hormones have receptors all over the body, not just in the organs they're designed to look after," says Dr Gribbin.

Menarche – your first period – typically occurs one and a half to three years after thelarche. During this time, oestrogen and progesterone have been acting progressively on the ovaries and uterus, ensuring they're big and robust enough to take care of that literally bloody business. "Fun fact," says Dr Gribbin, "when your periods start, you don't ovulate for another six to nine months." This failure to release an egg is known as anovulation. At this stage of puberty it's normal, but it can also happen later in life and is considered one of the leading causes of infertility.

Meanwhile, the GnRHs stimulate the ovaries to produce oestradiol, which in turn prompts the development of secondary sex characteristics, such as fat redistribution onto the hips and breasts. "The way fat is distributed in your body changes," says Dr Gribbin. "When you're an eight-year-old stick-thin little girl, your breasts might be about to start making a move, your nipples might start to change. But over the next four to six years, your weight will start going into different places. We're all born with the same number of fat cells we'll have all our life. But the fat distribution starts to change in puberty. That's based on growth hormone, insulin and oestrogen. And it goes round the hips on girls." It's also responsible for girls developing a broader pelvic bone, one designed to better facilitate childbirth; and for a change in the volume of our ovaries, from around $0.5cm^3$ to around $4cm^3$.

Oestrogen will refashion your uterus, changing it from a prepubertal tubular shape to a chunkier, pregnancy-accommodating pear shape; while your vulva will uh... I wanna say "enjoy"? Oh, why not!... Your vulva will *enjoy* an enlargement of the labia majora – the outer lips – and the labia minora, the inner, smaller, flaps, which extend down from the tip of the clitoris.

Why, I ask Dr Gribbin, does puberty feel so dramatic and intense and... violent, really? If it's so structured, so regimented, why does it feel so wild, so out of control?

"Brain development sort of speeds up. An emotionally very stable eight- or nine-year-old kid can become very labile during puberty."

Labile?

"It's a great word. Because it's not that they [teenagers] become unstable... It just means 'fluctuating, unreliable'. *Hormonal!*"

But normal?

"Completely normal. Some hormones can leave you feeling out of control. Especially adrenaline, which can sometimes spike just because something unexpected has happened. That then feeds back to your other hormones: your insulin, your cortisol especially. And neurological pathways are being laid down! I'm trying to remember what the specific pathway is called..."

Don't worry, I say. I'm going to zoom a neuroscientist.

PUBERTY AND THE FEMALE BRAIN

I wake up at 6am for a video call with neuroscientist Dr Sarah McKay – she's at her home in Sydney, and I'm in London, navigating the time difference. Despite the early hour, it proves entirely worthwhile, because she is *amazing*. I spend the following week resenting having to speak to people who *aren't* neuroscientists; I can't shake the feeling they're not worth it. Normos don't know anything cool about brains.

Dr McKay is an Oxford-educated New Zealander, an academic now based in Australia where she runs Think Brain, a science communications business that translates neuroscience so that businesses might better understand and apply it. Her particular area of interest is what happens to our brains when we go through different life phases, specifically puberty, pregnancy and menopause. It's an area she's researched and continues to research, tirelessly. She's analysed the brain scans of girls and women as they go through those life phases and written definitive books on the subject (among them, *The Woman's Brain Book* in 2018).

So, just wondering: what are our brains, like, made of? I say (by way of a casual opening gambit).

Dr McKay laughs, pauses, boggles – presumably as the true extent of the limits of my knowledge dawns on her.

"Gosh. Is that the actual question?

Yes.

"I've never been asked that before!"

God love the woman – she rolls with it.

"OK. Brains are made up of 86 billion neurons…"

Neurons = the basic units of the brain and the nervous system, the bricks of their houses, the grains of sand on their respective beaches. According to the University of Queensland, "they're responsible for receiving sensory input from the external world, for sending motor commands to our muscles, and for transforming and relaying the electrical signals at every step in between."

Neuron

"...and a whole lot of other billions of supporting cells," Dr McKay continues. "We've understood, for quite a long time, what neurons do. They communicate electrically, but also chemically, via synapses. The point-to-point connection between neurons is a synapse." This is a microscopic gap. "We've understood over time how those 86 billion neurons come together to communicate our thoughts, our feelings and our behaviours, and we're starting to understand what the support cells do. We used to think they were a bit like glue or scaffold, but we're understanding they play a role as well."

So we could think of the brain as a collection of 86 billion miniscule units that interact with each other constantly, and in doing so, make us move and think and feel. That make us *everything we are.* How amazing.

"I've been thinking it was amazing since I was 18," Dr McKay says. "I'm nearly 50 now. Every day, I still think it's the coolest thing ever."

My next question is a dangerous one, the kind considered by some to be profoundly problematic. Elements of the feminist movement consider its very existence "neurosexist", and believe it should simply not be asked. All it does, they argue, is reinforce stifling, poisonous gender stereotypes, primarily the idea that women are inherently inferior.

But it's also a question which has intrigued philosophers and scientists from the ancient Greeks on, plus it *really* fascinates me. So I ask it: is there a male brain and a female brain?

"That's the big question. It's really difficult to answer in a really short way. You have to be slightly long-winded."

Fine by me.

"We have biological males and biological females, and many aspects of our bodies, our nervous systems, our brains – which are part of our bodies – are very very similar, if not identical. We've got fingers and fingernails and hands and bones. And skin and hair and eyeballs that see, and legs that move us around the world, and hearts and digestive tracts… but there are also many aspects of our biology that are very very different.

"That's what enables there to be two biological species, which can reproduce. Evolution has selected for there to be two completely different biological sexes: male and female.

"And we understand that there are differences in terms of chromosomes, reproductive systems, in terms of secondary sex characteristics which emerge at puberty, in terms of genitals. And then there are other factors that overlap a whole lot…" Dr McKay goes on to tell me about something called "bimodal distribution". This is a set of data showing variation between two groups of people. She gave the example of height.

"I'm actually quite tall, and I have a very tall sibling. My sibling is six foot tall – taller than the average bloke – but that's my sister. She's a very, very tall woman."

Me too! I say. Both my siblings are taller than I am, maybe not taller than the average bloke, but probably getting there – and both are women. (The younger one, who is tallest of us all, was for some years of the opinion there should be some sort of law – at the very least, widely accepted and vigorously enforced etiquette – on shorter women not dating taller men, leaving them to taller women who, she felt, had fewer options.)

"And we kind of understand that there's average heights of men and there's average heights of women," Dr McKay continues, "but there's lots of overlap between the two – we can talk about average differences here, but we intuitively understand you can have really short dudes, and really tall women. There's a bit of a sex difference there in height: but there's also a ton of overlap."

Morpheus: I know bimodal distribution.

"Then, we start to look at behaviours. Let's talk about something silly, like knitting. Who likes to knit? Actually, one of the people I know who is the most prolific knitter, and has been ever since I've known him, is a Canadian bloke I went to university with. So: 'Do men like knitting? Do women like knitting? Are men better knitters than women?'"

Dr McKay tells me that she thinks of our brains as a reflection of the whole of our bodies; so much of them is neither male nor female. You could not, she says, crack upon the skull of a man, or a woman, "and go: 'Oh look, the ladies have got the pink brains! The gentlemen have got the blue brains!' They are bimodal."

Men's brains do tend to be around 10% bigger than women's on average, not because they're more intelligent – although from the 19th century on, when that size difference was first recognised, various scientists have attempted to use it as proof of just that – but rather, because it's necessary to drive a body which is, on average, bigger.

This is not the only difference, Dr McKay tells me. There are some parts of the brain where there is sexual dimorphism, a difference in appearance between males and females. "There's still a bit of overlap, but there's differences. Women have a special neurocircuitry that's involved with ovulation – obviously men don't have that. Men *do* have similar circuitry that's involved in regulating testosterone production, getting feedback on testosterone production from the testes."

I get it: because brains are fantastically complex, it takes an infinitely more complex kind of question to establish what we even mean by "a male brain" and "a female brain". Are we talking about anatomy, physiology, behaviour?

"Or network connections," Dr McKay says. "Are we talking about five-year-old boys and girls? Are we talking about kids going through puberty? Are we talking about a woman going through pregnancy versus a man of the same age? We have to start asking much more precise questions. We have to start asking: 'What is the difference that we are interested in? And how different is that difference?' Because there's a lot of overlap."

Now: puberty.

Brain development in puberty is triggered, I learn, by the same mechanism that triggers the development of our bodies – that surge in sex hormone, that turning-on of the hypothalamus, which pings a chemical message from our brain to our ovaries and uterus, prompting our breasts and pubic hair to grow.

"Brains have got receptors for sex hormones too," says Dr McKay. "Male brains and female brains follow the same trajectory: it's almost like they just have a different key to turn on the same car. But they end up in the same place, through pubertal development. So just think about it as brains are going through puberty too. There's a significant neurological transition taking place in teenagers' brains, driven by pubertal hormones."

And it's oestrogen and progesterone for girls, and testosterone for boys – though everyone has all three hormones, just in varying amounts.

"Yes."

First, we need to consider how the structure of our brains change in response to that surge in sex hormone. During childhood, our brains get gradually bigger, reaching near-adult size when we're around seven or eight. Although they won't get any larger in puberty – they couldn't, or they'd burst out of our skulls, apparently – they do still change, structurally; their ratios change.

Dr McKay starts casting around her desk for something.

"Uh… where's my brain?"

She produces a full-size plastic model of a brain.

"Here it is. Right. Grey matter is this wrinkly outer coating." She swirls her hand around those fat, juicy wormy, prominent ridges and the rivulets that divide them.

It's wrinkly like that, to pack more of it in, right? I say.

"Yeah! You can stuff more into an enclosed space. Like, if you've got a piece of paper and you scrunch it up."

I choose not to alert Dr McKay to the fact that I know this because it came up in an episode of the gorgeous, coincidentally Australian, comedy *Colin from Accounts*, during which, the main character, medical student Ashley, claimed that if all those wrinkles were ironed out flat, the brain would have the circumference of a 20" pizza.[6]

If grey matter is the wrinkly scrunched-up stuff on the outside of the brain, white matter is located deeper within, and is the means by which its different regions are connected. They're wires, highways, axons, says Dr McKay. When the brain is developing in puberty, grey matter has been observed to get thinner. This may sound alarming, as if it were degenerating. In fact, it's the opposite. That thinning of grey matter allows for slicker interconnection;

---

6   Sadly, and despite some effort, I've been unable to verify this.

it's a streamlining process, a sharpening-up.

The parts of the brain that are subject to this thinning and sharpening are incredibly significant. They're the areas which, in puberty "are undergoing critical periods of experience-dependent development. We see the emergence of a kind of *mastery* of skills, improvement of the types of functions that those singular brain regions are involved with."

What are we talking about, when we say teenagers need "experience-dependent development"? Social and emotional development. Your teenage years are classically the time during which your focus turns outwards, away from your family, towards your friends. I remember voraciously seeking out those friendship tribes, those identities and the people associated with them, trying on goth and indie kid and Wham! fan and skater girl for size. All those sharply delineated microcultures, all offering a framework, a sense of belonging and new thrilling horizons, all at once. All of them, apparently, a consequence of the way in which my brain was changing shape.

"Your brain is driven to belong to a new tribe. There's an evolutionary reason [for that]: you want to find a mate from... Well, not from your family."

Reasonable.

Yet along with that brain-inspired compulsion to seek out newness, new people, new situations, comes a kicker of a payback, which is also a consequence of how your brain changes shape in puberty. It suddenly becomes incredibly sensitive to social experiences, even as it drives you to seek them out. This is all due to a thinning of the grey matter in parts of the brain involved in social cognition, which, according to Dr McKay is "thinking about what other people are thinking. Thinking about what other people are feeling. Reading facial expressions. Picking up social cues."

This, then, is why we feel so incredible raw and sensitive as teenagers, so awkward and inclined to overanalyse, so ready to conclude that everyone hates us, that the world is against us, that we're unpopular and unlovable and destined to live our lives out, miserable and quite alone.

It's a painful, and, according to neuroscience, necessary, part of the process.

"Because your brain is in this exquisite state of readiness to learn, all these social experiences you have are so meaningful, but that also comes with vulnerability," says Dr McKay.

Which, you'd think, would be quite enough for one individual teetering on the brink of adulthood to deal with, but oh no! A higher-order part of our brain – our cerebral cortex, an outer layer that runs along the top of it, and is responsible for things like language, memory, reason, decision-making, and (in this case, crucially) emotion – is also evolving. During puberty, our brain is grasping its way towards a state of being able to regulate emotions better, contain them, contextualise them. To elucidate this point, Dr McKay gives this example:

"You're 48. You walk into a room and everyone's laughing. You go: 'Ah, they're probably laughing at some joke.' When you're 15, you're: 'Oh my God oh my God oh my God they're laughing at me, I'm going to go away and cry!'"

Which is funny because it's true, but also, really not funny at all. I can remember it so clearly, that desperate self-consciousness, that deep conviction I was perpetually a hair's breadth, or the wrong type of eyeliner, or an involuntary hiccup, or (God forbid) public fart away from destroying the tissue-thin, ultra-tenuous grasp I did have on the meagre social standing I'd achieved at secondary school. The regrettable lengths I'd go to, to ensure another day passed at the coalface of teenagehood without me taking a deep dive into social pariahdom (up to and including how uproariously I laughed when a male friend said to a female friend: "But you're not paranoid, Carly! Everyone really does hate you!") How awful I felt when everyone but me was invited to a classmate's birthday trip to a roller-rink, which he'd later insist was an administrative error, but was it?

It is, by anyone's measure, a vast amount to deal with, yet the outward expression of this remodelling that the teenage brain undergoes is mocked and dismissed and belittled by... adults who've been through it so know exactly how painful it is.

"When a baby learns to talk, and a baby learns to walk, they stumble and fall," says Sarah McKay. "They make mistakes, mispronounce things, because their brains are in a state of neuroplasticity. Unfortunately, we tend to dismiss teenagers when they're going through this. When a toddler falls over, we don't go: 'Look at them! They haven't even learned to walk yet! They probably won't learn to walk properly until they're FOUR!' We're really mean to teenagers, and supportive of toddlers. We need to think about how we can support these brains as they're going through these learning processes. That's what the brain's doing; it's trying its hardest to learn, to make its way in this world as it's becoming an adult."

Yet another consequence of grey matter thinning in puberty is an increased propensity for taking risks. Experimenting with drugs, lying to your parents about your whereabouts because they wouldn't let you do the thing you were hell-bent on doing, were you to tell them the truth, driving far too fast in cars you barely know how to manoeuvre… Although, as Dr McKay says, there are plenty of other social risks you can take. "You take risks putting your hand up in the classroom, volunteering an idea everyone else might disagree with. That's a big risk too." It is, she tells me, about learning how far you can take things, and who you are in this adult world. I quietly remember the time a friend and I ducked out of school at lunchtime, an activity that was strictly forbidden according to school rules, to meet a couple of boys from a nearby private school, an activity that was socially *verboten* according to the lore governing the separation of private and state school kids around my way, circa 1986. Our intended assignation was somehow "discovered" by boys from our school, who became outraged by the possibility that we – two girls they'd known for years, in whom they'd shown precisely zero romantic interest previously – were being pursued by boys other than them; posh boys at that! They tracked us down at our meeting, an actual physical scuffle entailed, and one of the private school boys acquired a bloody nose, over which, I felt terribly guilty. That was the last time my friend and I ever saw them. The raging boys from our school, meanwhile, reverted to having absolutely zero interest in either of us, in the aftermath of this unfortunate episode.

This kind of risk-taking behaviour classically peaks in the mid-teen years, then tapers off, as we get older. It's interesting from a neuroscientific perspective, I learn, because, as Dr McKay tells me, "Teenagers have the ability to make smart decisions when they're alone. Typically, what they do is make the decisions which can get them in trouble because they're looking for – what matters more than anything – tribe acceptance! They don't usually drive a car fast when they're on their own, or when their dad's next to them. But they'll drive stupidly when their mates are there. Their mates are bigging them on, and what matters more is not the potential danger, but their mates."

YOUNG WOMEN AND MENTAL HEALTH

There's a question that pops up, over and over, as I feel my way forward on this gig. I try and ignore it, deny it, brush it aside for later, but it crops up again and again, as a side note in studies of hormones, fertility and addiction, as a consequence of bad period pain, and so on and so forth.

The question is this: is having a female body bad for our mental health?

The early indications are that the state of being a woman definitely is. A report by the British Medical Association[7] found that in 2016, one in five adult women, compared with one in eight adult men, had a common mental health disorder – depression or anxiety – and that those trends were largely overall stable for men, though rapidly increasing in women. The same report found that young women were particularly at risk, and that one in five women between the ages of 16 and 25 reported recent self-harm. In 2020, a UK government study into the gender differences in mental health found women reporting greater incidences of anxiety and depression, major stress relating to their finances and major stress relating to Covid-19 (which was

---

7 Addressing unmet needs in women's mental health, *BMA*, 2018, https://www.bma.org.uk/media/2115/bma-womens-mental-health-report-aug-2018.pdf

running rampant, at the time of the study).[8]

Although men are three times more likely to commit suicide than women (suicide is the biggest killer of men under 50, according to mental health charity Mind),[9] women are more likely to have suicidal thoughts, and more likely to attempt suicide. A study published in 2022 by the *British Journal of General Practice* found that between 2003 and 2018, women were twice as likely as men to be prescribed medications to relieve the symptoms of anxiety.

But why? Is this conditioning? Circumstantial? Is it because women tend to shoulder more domestic pressure – housework, care for children or ageing relatives – in addition to work pressure? Is it because society compels us to shoot for perfection in all areas of our lives, which can only lead to burnout and feelings of failure? Is it hormonal? Neural? Is it just that we're better at expressing ourselves and asking for help, so we're skewing the figures by virtue of speaking up?

I definitely need to talk to a psychologist; and, given that a study by the Mental Health Foundation suggests that "50% of mental health problems are established by the age of 14, 75% by the age of 24",[10] I definitely need to talk to one who specialises in young people.

---

8 COVID-19 mental health and wellbeing surveillance: gender spotlight, GOV. UK, 2021 – https://www.gov.uk/government/publications/covid-19-mental-health-and-wellbeing-surveillance-spotlights/gender-covid-19-mental-health-and-wellbeing-surveillance-report

9 Mental health facts and statistics, Mind, 2020 – https://www.mind.org.uk/information-support/types-of-mental-health-problems/statistics-and-facts-about-mental-health/how-common-are-mental-health-problems/

10 Children and young people: statistics, Mental Health Foundation – https://www.mentalhealth.org.uk/explore-mental-health/statistics/children-young-people-statistics

Dr Tara Porter is a clinical psychologist, therapist and a writer who has worked for over 20 years in the eating disorders unit of Child and Adolescent Mental Health Services (CAMHS) in London and, consequently, she tells me when we meet in my local branch of Gail's, "I've spoken to hundreds of teenage girls about their bodies." Her 2022 book *You Don't Understand Me: The Young Woman's Guide to Life*, is a *Sunday Times* bestseller; by the time I've finished this one, she's written another, *Good Enough: Break free from the perfection trap and raise happy, self-reliant children*.

She is considered and calm, and she teases me for my repeated attempts to spin her words into grabby, splashy headlines.

I start by verifying that girls really do suffer poorer mental health.

"What we know is, teenage girls make up the majority of the increase in referrals that we've seen in CAMHS services."

I ask if this has always been the case, because: it certainly feels like it – doesn't it? All the things I instinctively thought I knew, all the things I'd heard and seen for… well, the whole of my life, really; certainly long before I started any formal research into the subject; all of it, the anecdotal, the observed, the first-hand experience, *everything* suggests that women and girls experience poorer mental health than boys and men. So have women and girls always been less mentally healthy? Dr Porter says that, when she digs into the figures, the raw data, she always sees a huge split between girls and boys. "Whether that means more girls are suffering than boys – I'm not sure. They're suffering with things like depression and anxiety – but boys are suffering too. We certainly know that from the statistics on suicide. There are lots of men that, I think, are silently suffering." Alternatively, she says, the fact that male depression and anxiety are expressed as anger and aggression might explain why many more boys than girls are currently being supported by council-run organisations, the police and probation services, who are all trying to help keep them away from criminality.

"The short answer," Dr Porter continues, "would be: yes, many more girls and women get diagnosed with depression and anxiety. But it's more complicated and nuanced than that."

According to Dr Porter, there is currently "a perfect storm" driving the poor mental health of teenage girls and young women. Social media is one part of it; and psychologists are trying to unpack precisely why and how it's causing so much harm. "There are quite a lot of studies about the impact of viewing so-called 'perfect bodies,'" she says, wrapping finger quotes around the words, to show how bogus the concept is to her, "on your idea of *your* body." All the evidence so far is overwhelmingly – unsurprisingly – that the viewing of "fitspiration" bodies online, of bodies trained, then electronically altered and filtered, to look as toned and honed and unbothered by cellulite, hair and blemishes as possible, makes those looking at them feel less satisfied with their own.

Does that relate to boys and girls, young men as well as young women? I ask.

"That research is done mainly on girls," Dr Porter tells me, "Some preliminary studies suggest that it might be true for men too, but it does seem that women are exposed to more images then men."

Does she think it's definitive?

"When I read that research, it's not the kind of thing where you're thinking: there's two sides to this story. Overall, the majority of the research shows this."

In addition to which, social media has been shown to interfere with many of the things known to support good mental health. It disrupts sleep, keeps people indoors (when being outside is demonstrably beneficial to our mood) and limits the amount of time we spend with real people, in real life, as opposed to having fleeting, less emotionally rewarding connections with them online.

Dr Porter believes that it's the comparison and competition aspect of social media that is really toxic. It only seems to benefit mental health when people use it creatively, or to make connections.

Is there some psychological trait that makes some people more or less likely to use social media in a healthy way? I'm only asking because I've had a rough old time of it, on Twitter in particular in the past – me! A fully grown adult whose brain developed in puberty without being subject to social media or the internet, the demands and comparisons and potential for bullying that come with that – because it hadn't been invented at that point, and yet, I have still suffered. Very nearly crashed and burned at one point, when a wave of social media ire crashed down over me in response to something I'd published. And I, then in my early 40s, stopped eating and sleeping, and found myself consumed by a level of anxiety I'd never known before, and also, by pure *shame*. But – was that about me? Might a different person have bounced through it cheerfully?

"Interesting question. I don't know. I know from patients, if you have a tendency towards anxiety and depression, [social media] can really spiral that tendency."

I've heard anxiety described (probably on some Instagram post, oh the irony!) as being rooted in fear of the future, while depression is a preoccupation with the past. Dr Porter agrees (at least) that anxiety is generally a worry about what's going to happen.

"So if you're thinking: 'I'm not going to pass my exams, I'm not going to amount to anything, I'm never going to get a job…' being on social media can really spiral that. You're looking for confirmation, evidence." And social media, viewed with anxious eyes, is precisely that. For example, if an anxious young person, building up to an exam, convinced they're not working hard enough, and constantly monitoring online the activities of friends also working towards that exam, sees a post stating: "I worked for five hours today", when they've only done four, it can really throw them. They immediately think their friend's going to do better than them, and it's a downward spiral. "Competition and comparison drives anxiety," says Dr Porter.

This, I learn, is particularly the case with teenage girls. Dr Porter tells me that girls tend to use the internet and social media in a very different way from teenage boys. Boys mainly game, while girls connect socially – a social connection that leads to competition, negative comparison, judgement.

"I was doing a talk at a school recently, a girls' school, which is next door to a boys' school. Afterwards, the assistant head was walking me out, and he said something which really resonated, something about the way girls have friendships. He told me that when he stands looking down into these two playgrounds on these two secondary schools, he looks at the girls, and he looks at the boys – and what do you think the girls are doing?"

I sigh, because I don't even have to think about the answer. I know. I have been a teenage girl.

They're standing in groups, talking, I tell Dr Porter.

"And what are the boys doing?" she asks me.

They're playing.

"Right."

Girls, she explains, connect through sharing an emotional space, a mental space. Their friendships are based on talking. "They're in each other's minds, they know what each other is thinking, they're thinking about the same thing, whatever that is." Boys, meanwhile, connect by doing something together. "They don't sit there and talk about it. They game." This is the process by which girls end up internalising their pain, while boys externalise it.

"Girls turn it inside – they don't feel good enough or thin enough. Fit enough. Clever enough. Popular enough."

So these narratives, these notions, these *clichés*, really, which I've always believed about the respective mental health of teenage girls and boys, young women and young men, seem to be borne out by the considerable experience of mental health professionals; and exacerbated by social media.

But *why*? Is this societal? Hormonal? Does testosterone somehow drive the desire to game, to externalise pain; oestrogen or progesterone the desire to compare, and to internalise pain? I had found a report that suggests that the reason women cry more than men might be because prolactin – the breast-feeding hormone – promotes crying, while testosterone inhibits it.

Might there then be some degree of hormonal influence, or just *something*, about our bodies, or our brains, that means women have less good mental health?

"I've been a psychologist for 26 years, and it's always been true that girls internalise, and boys externalise – even before social media," says Dr Porter. She goes on to explain how both nature and nurture might be at play. While girls are taught by society to connect, it's possible some characteristics or preferences are innate. She gives the example from her own experience of bringing up her children.

"As soon as my [elder] son could pick anything up, he picked up a ball. He wanted to *do*. I was bringing them up in a gender-neutral, north London, liberal way: he had a pushchair and a kitchen as well. But he gravitated towards doing. So there seems to be something a bit nature-y there as well." I think of my goddaughter and my nieces, of how ineluctably drawn they were, around the age of two, two and a half, to the colour pink, despite their parents' best efforts; of the row I had with my goddaughter over possession of a very gaudy, ultra-feminine, feather boa one Christmas Day when she was about four. I also remember reading an article a colleague wrote some decades ago about how she'd refused to buy her twin four-year-old sons "boy" toys, such as trucks and cars, or indulge gender stereotypes at any point, but had discovered them both biting their toast into the shape of guns, then using them to "shoot" each other, one breakfast.

However, Dr Porter thinks there is another factor in this perfect storm affecting girls' mental health, in addition to social media and genetics.

"There's something in parenting," she tells me, "and the way we've educated this last generation of kids, which is impacting mental health problems."

The concept of "parenting" as an active verb, she says, only evolved at the turn of this century. "Before that, people were just parents, they weren't 'parenting' in an active, outcome-focussed way. That older style of parenting is widely known as 'benign neglect', and relies on the idea that parents are bonded to their children through nature, so needn't really do much more than hope for the best for them and protect them from the most pressing, immediate expressions of danger... Giving kids a happy, good childhood. That's what I would hope, perhaps optimistically. That that was the best aim."

But things changed in the 21st century. Dr Porter gives another example from her personal experience. She remembers that when she had her eldest child in 2000, and she was looking through a brochure to pick some toys, she found that there were hardly any that were not educational. They all seemed to be geared towards providing children with opportunities for getting the best outcome. This, she thinks, is entirely symptomatic of a broader shift in ideas around raising and educating children. She points to an education system which is now infinitely more focussed on outcomes, on the "output" of individual children. "A generation ago, we didn't have league tables, for example." Now? Everything, and every child, is constantly rated and measured, and ranked in terms of peers. Parents have become extremely focussed on giving their kids opportunities, she says; and children can experience this as intense pressure. "Often what I hear reflected in the patients I see is a sense of 'everyone expects it of me. People will be disappointed in me.'"

At the same time, and by no coincidence, the education system has been redesigned, changing it into what Dr Porter describes as "an arms race. So we've gone from O level, where you could get a grade A, to GCSE where you can get an A*, to now, where the A* is getting subdivided into different degrees of excellence, the 8 and the 9… You've got the SATs in Year 6, in primary schools. Schools are graded by their SATs results."

SATs were introduced in the UK gradually between 1991 and 1998 to monitor the impact of the newly introduced national curriculum on education and to establish which schools were implementing it well. It had nothing whatsoever to do with grading the achievements of individual pupils – but now? "It's become something parents tutor their kids for. Primary schools send out revision booklets in the Easter holidays." Exams have therefore become part of the system by which children feel constantly and intensely tested and judged, which can only intensify the experience of an adolescence already shaped – corrupted, actually – by the pressures of comparison and competition.

The beginning of every school year, Dr Porter tells me, begins with the head of whichever year students find themselves in standing at the front of assembly and telling them: "This year is the most important year of your school career!" which, of course, can't possibly be true – it can only be one of them, by definition. But girls hear this, and think: "Oh right, I need to work harder than I've ever worked before." Boys, meanwhile, often disregard it, which can result in them becoming disenfranchised from education entirely.

We move on to eating disorders, Dr Porter's specialism. She was one of my very earliest interview subjects, the first to raise the issue of women, girls and our endlessly complex relationship with weight. But I hear it again and again and again, invoked in relation to addiction, pregnancy, infertility, menstrual cycles and menopause. Undereating and obesity – they're like evil twins pushing and pulling women, our bodies, our physical and mental health apart at the seams.

They are, Dr Porter tells me, much more prevalent in women and girls, who are far more likely to express their depression and anxiety by starving their bodies to fit into a societal standard. This is not to suggest boys are immune to disordered eating: they account for around 10% of cases. "For most boys puberty takes them closer to an idealised body shape – they get more masculine. The problem is in huge part the idealisation of a pre-pubertal body as a suitable body for grown women." Dr Porter tells me that, for a young pubertal woman, an eating disorder, which may have started as a way to manage their distress, can have the secondary gain for them of not having to deal with periods or sexualisation. It can take them back to the relative simplicity of childhood, where they didn't have to worry about sanitary protection or bras, or being cat-called in the street. This can seem better, at least at first, especially for a girl going through puberty before the rest of her peer group.

I learn that while mental health issues are increasing overall at a steady pace, eating disorders are rising at a much faster rate, relatively.

"I link that back to social media, the increased visual culture, and how much pressure there is to compare your own with other bodies," says Dr Porter. And although it's always important to have this validated by a highly qualified, practised and experienced professional, we knew this, didn't we? We knew it because we're more than aware of the impact social media is having on *us*, as adults; how endless exposure to rigorously curated and painstakingly filtered images of fitness instructors in luxe sports bras telling us we're not eating enough protein or lifting "heavy" enough have dented our sense of ourselves and our own bodies over the course of the last decade – *and we are adults whose brains formed without the pernicious influence of the internet.*

Dr Porter explains the mechanism by which eating disorders operate. They're not necessarily the starting point of mental health issues, merely an escalation of them, an attempt at managing emotional distress.

"What I'd see often is girls – and boys – showing distress through self-harm and suicidal action. They would show up at A&E having been discovered cutting themselves. They would get perhaps a seven-day follow-up appointment, then be put on a waiting list [for therapy]." Having arrived at a crisis point, but finding themselves in a waiting list limbo, they try to find other ways to deal with it.

Starving yourself? "Young people find when they don't eat, their feelings sometimes go away," says Dr Porter. Because, if you're starving yourself, if you're constantly consumed by hunger, you're *only* thinking about that. Your physical pain overrides your emotional pain. "In time, of course, the body pushes back, and wants to overeat to compensate. Some dieters then go on to binge eat or engage in patterns of bingeing and starving, so what starts off as a way to manage their feelings, in time spirals to make the whole situation much much worse." However, it can also expedite treatment, in the UK at least. In 2015, the government pledged a big increase in funding for child and adolescent eating-disorder services and targets have to be met, which means you are generally seen more quickly than other CAMH services, though it can vary depending on where you live. "When kids stop eating, they do get seen – so when young people are struggling with multiple 'conditions' the service they are picked up by first is often an eating disorder one."

I ask Dr Porter what she thinks is at the heart of all this female pain. "The core stress is not being good enough. Whether it's OCD [obsessive-compulsive disorder], depression, anxiety, eating disorders." They are overwhelmed by all the expectations and standards imposed on them, which they find impossible to meet.

What helps, she says, is being listened to and understood. Having someone bear witness to their distress. Different types of therapy, such as cognitive behavioural therapy and psychotherapy can help people to make sense of their situation and then change it.

Dr Porter is hopeful things will get better, that we'll get better at understanding our thinking around our bodies, for a start. She tells me this fascinating thing about how we see our bodies in the mirror: not how we *perceive* them, but literally, how our eyes see them. We always think we are shorter than we actually are, shorter than other people perceive us when they look at us, because we don't factor in the distance between us and the mirror.

"If you're six feet away, your reflection is half the [actual] size. But your eyes automatically make the adjustment. If you walk backwards and forwards, your size in the mirror will change, but you never notice that because you have object constancy."

Mirrors warp our idea of ourselves.

On top of which, selfie culture, the endless urge to compare the very worst ideas or pictures of ourselves with the very best, most carefully angled and filtered images of everyone else, serves to compound dangerously negative self-image.

But yes! Still Dr Porter is hopeful for better things to come.

"Every generation reacts against the excesses of the previous generation. I think my generation reacted against the benign neglect of our parents in the 70s, so gave our kids all these opportunities which have become embedded in their minds as expectations that they can't meet. I think our kids will react again. I think they'll do better on this. Like Philip Larkin said: 'They f*ck you up, your mum and dad.'"

WHAT I KNOW NOW

- Sex hormones are essential to how the female body works. They are predominantly oestrogen – the Beyoncé hormone, the party hormone, the hormone of confidence and (according to one study) infidelity – and progesterone – a stern, serious, risk-averse manager of oestrogen's excesses.

- Puberty is on a rigorously managed schedule. It begins when the female sex hormones get switched on by the brain; specifically, in the hypothalamus and the pituitary gland.

- Puberty remodels bodies – forming breasts, broadening hips, changing the shape of the uterus, as well as brains. Brains in puberty become painfully sensitive to social interaction, while also compelling their owners to seek it out.

- Male and female brains are the same, but different.

- Girls and women present with considerably more mental health issues than boys or men. This is in part because girls and women tend to internalise their emotional pain and blame themselves for it, while boys and men tend to externalise it, blaming others and acting aggressively towards them.

CHAPTER THREE

THE MENSTRUAL CYCLE

As I remember it, the biggest upheaval puberty dropped, uninvited, on my body, by far – the most tedious, gross, unwelcome, embarrassing, painful and difficult to manage logistically speaking, was (bloody, bloody) periods. (I find I still can't bring myself to say "my periods". It's an over-identification too far.)

Left to our own devices, I'm reasonably sure not a single one of us would opt for them, would we? If they were somehow optional, if our bodies could function perfectly well without their turmoil and drama? If they weren't also a teenage status symbol, a rite of passage, a passport into adulthood. *Oh God, it's all so complicated, isn't it?*

And yet, as ballet-obsessive Dr Nicky Keay puts it: "The most beautiful choreography of all the hormonal systems is that of the female menstrual cycle. Look at the timing of it!" She opens her book, *Hormones, Health and Human Potential* (2022), at page 94 and shows me the graph printed there. Four coloured lines swoop and soar and ebb and flow and glide and rebound off and around each other in pace with the 28-day scope of the average menstrual cycle (although menstrual cycles of anything from 23 to 35 days are considered to be within a "normal" range). They represent: oestradiol, progesterone, luteinising hormone (LH) and follicle-stimulating hormone (FSH – told you they'd start to feel familiar), and I concede, they do look dramatic and grace-ful and potent. You could definitely perceive it as dancing.

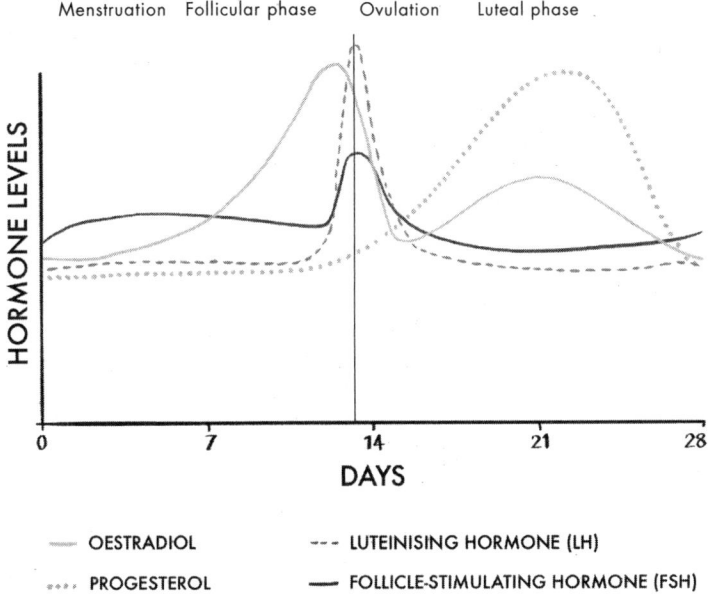

"Look at it!" Dr Keay says again. She's beaming, her face is all alight (and I smile too, because this woman's curious, obvious and somehow *pure* love of hormones is quite contagious).

Do we have more hormones than men?

"We have more *interesting* hormones, let's be honest. But because they change a lot, that's where the challenge is, for our mental and physical health. It's why they work. But it is where the challenge is. And every woman is slightly different, which is the other crucial thing. Slightly different levels, slightly different timings. People will have an individual biological response. Some women have premenstrual syndrome (PMS), some women don't, for example. Even with the same level of progesterone. I get a bit frustrated when I see [women] blaming hormones, making out we're somehow… fighting against them."

We aren't?

"No!"

"We talk about 'balancing your hormones'. Listen: hormones know quite well how to balance themselves. They've had millions of years of evolution, they know what to do."

"Hippocrates – Greek chap, 2000 years ago – said the surest way to health: just the right amount of exercise, just the right amount of nourishment – not too little, not too much."

By "the surest way to health", do you mean to well-functioning hormones?

"Yes. I'd add stress management and sleep. But yes."

Here's what I thought a menstrual cycle involved before I met Dr Keay: there are days when we're not having a period, when basically nothing happens; days when we feel like crap because we're *about* to have a period (trembling on its precipitous brink like scratchy, crotchety, wobbly, raging, whimpering lemmings); days when we feel a different kind of crap (and a whole lot of pain) because we *are* having a period; and the day its stops and we're back to nothing happening, rinse (our knickers, generally) and repeat.[11]

---

11 The one other thing I think I know about the menstrual cycle is that a group of women living or working in close proximity over an extended period of time will "sync", start having their periods at the same time, although, it turns out, I don't actually know this at all, because it isn't true. "It was suggested," says Dr Keay, "but reviewing in detail seems to show that a group of women together for some time (e.g. at boarding school), [merely] by chance would have some synchronicity."

According to Dr Keay and her graph, however, it is rather more complicated than no period, period. A lot happens, hormonally speaking – and it is happening *all the time*.

The menstrual cycle, as this graph shows it, is divided into four distinct phases of hormonal activity, all of which are driven by the hypothalamus and the pituitary gland (of course they are).

The phases are:

Days 1–5 (ish) – menstruation, during which, oestradiol, progesterone and LH levels are pretty much flatlining, though FSH levels are higher, riding at about 35% of their full potential; they've been on a gradual rise since around Day 25 of the previous cycle. It is this plummeting in hormones, in particular this withdrawal from progesterone, that causes the lining of the womb to fall away and leave your body, in the form of a period.

The follicular phase – which begins around Day 6, and lasts until Days 12–13, during which LH and progesterone snooze on – this is just not their time – oestradiol cranks up, slowly, slowly, a cable car in the early phase of ascent, and FSH rises further yet, peaking at 60–70% of its full extent – around Day 7–8, before sloping off gently once again. FSH is produced by the pituitary to stimulate follicles – teeny tiny little waggly finger-type things – on the surface of the ovaries, one of which will mature an egg (usually one, occasionally more), basically readying it for fertilisation, then pregnancy.

Ovulation, Days 13, 14, 15 (ish) – when oestradiol, LH and FSH suddenly shoot right up to the top of the graph, to the peak of their potential. This is when the egg, matured through the follicular phase, is released from the ovary, and moves along the fallopian tube, aided by muscular contractions and cilia, microscopic hair-like structures which vibrate *and* have adhesive properties (how fancy), towards the uterus. Should it encounter a sperm along its way, that egg may become fertilised.

The luteal phase, Days 16–28 (ish); when oestradiol falls away, then curves up again (much more gently than it did pre-ovulation) around Day 21, *then* slopes off on a downward curve. LH drops away completely, FSH dwindles downwards from its initial ovulation high, then starts ticking up again around Day 25. Progesterone, meanwhile, runs the show, dominating proceedings – you've got almost twice as much of it in your system as you do oestradiol by Day 21, which, as Dr Keay points out, makes sense. "Think about it. Progesterone = 'pro-gestation'. Your body is behaving as if it's pregnant [even if it isn't]." Progesterone makes the lining of your uterus thicken so that, assuming an egg *was* fertilised during its travels along the fallopian tube, it might embed itself in it and start growing into a baby. If that doesn't happen, if no egg has been fertilised, then, around Day 26 or 27 (with a cycle length between 21 and 35 days considered normal), progesterone drops off completely, along with LH and oestradiol… And we're back to menstruation again, Day 1.

Menstruation is the result of the falling levels of progesterone. This fall in progesterone is accompanied by production in the womb lining of mediators (messengers) of inflammation. The best known of these are prostaglandins (NB: these are not a type of progesterone as progesterone is a steroid hormone and prostaglandins are not). This "natural" inflammation in the womb lining at the time of menstruation each month is coupled with the shedding of the womb lining, although we still need a better understanding of all the pieces of this complex jigsaw. Production in the womb muscle of prostaglandins at the time of the period may also causes contractions and cramps.

The discarded womb lining is ejected from your bod in the form of blood and goopy, stringy tissue, a process which, yep, as we've said, takes an average of five days – though can take as few as two, or as many as eight – and tends to be heaviest for the first 48 hours, and to involve the loss of somewhere between one and five tablespoons of blood, although many women lose much more (and I'll come back to that, cos it's important, under-recognised, much more common than I, at least, had appreciated – and generally pretty unforgivably, unacceptably sh*t).

So that's the *actual* menstrual cycle. A meticulously choreographed push and pull and rise and fall of four main hormones; hormones that are constantly in motion, because, as Dr Keay explains, hormones need to fluctuate to work. "It's like sport, or exercise: if you do exactly the same thing [all the time], the body gets bored. If you give it exactly the same level of oestrogen all the time, where's the light and shade? It doesn't know what the high was, what the low was, the receptors get bored, think there's nothing to do. It's the change that's important."

HORMONES AND BEHAVIOUR

But what do those changes mean, in terms of how we experience life? I've spent decades cycling through these rigid, proscriptive hormonal patterns, decades swirling around in 'em, an internal, eternal washing-machine programme; yet never properly – or even, improperly, perfunctorily – stopped to think about what they might mean to me in terms of their impact on my emotions, my behaviour, my personality or my ability to perform. I mean, *obviously* I knew about PMS, pre-menstrual syndrome. *Obviously* I knew the edginess and foul temper that blows in like a sea squall two-ish days before my period, although sometimes it's more bleak, just *sad*, and it's always characterised by the inar-guable certainty that I am, after all, just rubbish. Pointless. Unat-tractive. Crap at my job. Unpleasant company. Et cetera. Did I know I was in the dying days of my luteal phase and experienc-ing a response to a sudden, dramatic drop in progesterone, accompanied by very low levels of oestrogen, so, basically in a hormonal withdrawal, which was determining my mood? No. Of course I didn't. But I did certainly recognise that recurring pattern early on in adult life; came to understand it as a passing phase, learned to apply coping techniques accordingly (even if they were only taking myself away from the world and sulking).

But, given what I know now about the hormonal upheaval in play at *all* other points in the menstrual cycle, given I've seen it on Dr Keay's chart, might it follow that an equivalent awareness of what that means, how it might feel, how it might be under-stood, navigated and managed, just as my PMS is (kinda) under-stood, navigated and managed… Might that be, oh, I don't know: illuminating? Enlightening? Arguably: absolutely essen-tial intelligence?

Absolutely, according to Maisie Hill, menstrual coach, midwife, birth doula, whom I track down after seeing her bestselling book – *Period Power* (2019) – for sale in the reception area of the Pilates studio I frequent. I google Hill, and discover she's routinely referred to as "The Womb Whisperer", as her area of particular interest is how we feel and act at any given point in our menstrual cycle, how those feelings and actions are informed by our hormones and how we can manage them. Hill has spent over 15 years coaching women on their menstrual cycles, through their pain and their moods and their crashing self-doubt. She's worked with hundreds and hundreds of us, observed us, as we dance this infernal, majestic dance with our own body chemistry, noted the similarities and individualities, the wild variations and hilarious, beautiful peculiarities in menstrual cycles.

It's all so very far up My Alley, so I instantly send her an email and arrange an interview.

Maisie Hill joins our Zoom, apologises for being (minutes, if that) late, explains she was having a horse-riding lesson (the best reason for a little lateness I've encountered since Johnny Depp went AWOL on our interview appointment in Cannes for 48 hours. His reason? Kate Moss). Hill is flamingly red-haired and unflinchingly direct, with the most captivating tattoos up and down her arm and onto her fingers: the kind that make me itch to get something similar myself.

She tells me that the star of the menstrual cycle show is ovulation.

I see. Should it really be called the Ovulation Cycle?

"Perhaps, but let's not confuse things."

OK.

"But when we're talking about the ebb and flow of hormones, on a very simple level: when your periods start, your hormone levels are very low."

Because their levels have been slipping away since ovulation, halfway through our cycle?

"Yes."

And that's why we *feel* so low when our periods start? Hormones low = us, feeling low?

"Some people do. Some people don't. It's not just about where your hormone levels are in the cycle; it's also about your hormone levels within that part of the cycle and the relationship between that hormone and other hormones. And then, it's also about your sensitivity and response to those hormones, which is all about neurotransmitters."

Neurotransmitters are not unlike hormones: they are chemical substances released by the brain, which zoom off towards receptors, which then act on their instructions. Unlike hormones, they are not released from the brain into the bloodstream to travel to other parts of the body. Neurotransmitters only ever zap from one part of the brain to another. They move between "synaptic clefts", which are the spaces between neurons; they control many things, but high among them is mood. See serotonin and dopamine – neurotransmitters associated with mood management, the experience of pleasure, satisfaction and motivation; also endorphin, which when released, binds with pain receptors in the brain to relieve pain, reduce stress and fatigue and even negative thoughts, which is why exercise – a key trigger of endorphins – is so, so very good for your head, as well as your body... But that's for another day.

Neurotransmitters have an impact on sex hormones, and vice versa; the two interact to determine your mood. Oestrogen, for example, has been shown to increase synthesis of dopamine; according to a study from the University of Yale, oestrogen deprivation leads to the death of dopamine cells in the brain,[12] which, the study proposed, is why Parkinson's disease is more common in men than it is pre-menopausal women, but then increases in women after menopause, when oestrogen supplies are diminished.

------

12 Estrogen deprivation leads to death of dopamine cells in the brain, Yale University, *ScienceDaily*, 2000 – www.sciencedaily.com/releases/2000/12/001204072446.htm

"For some people, that low hormone state at the start of a period can feel like a relief," Hill goes on, "if, pre-menstrually, you've got quite severe mood symptoms happening: irritability, rage, depression. Whereas for others, they can feel like they haven't got the verbal recall that they have at other times, for example. When your hormones are at the start of the cycle, you maybe feel a bit vulnerable, a bit raw, a bit exposed. Not as up for things."

Is that because we're very low on oestrogen – aka, the Up For It hormone, the Beyoncé hormone (as Hill herself has been known to refer to it), liquid mojo (as I'm beginning to think of it) – at that point, so early in our cycle?

"Yes."

And what does it feel like to you?

"Like: 'Oh! I'm back in the room!' I can start off feeling, around the time of my period, like I want to rest more. That doesn't necessarily mean lying down; just easing off. Once that oestrogen starts to drip in, it's like my brain fires up, my body fires up, and we're off! And then, that starts increasing day by day, a gradual influence… It peaks a couple of days before ovulation, and that's when we've also got testosterone showing up."

To recap, women do have the male sex hormone testosterone, just, typically, in much smaller levels than men. While it's the primary sex hormone in men, responsible for the development and maintenance of testicles, prostate, muscle mass, and body hair; in both men and women it's associated with mood, cognition, sexual behaviour, metabolism, energy and bone density. In women, testosterone is produced by our ovaries. We generally have around 0.5–1.5nmol/L in our system, while men have around 8–29nmol/L. According to Dr Nicky Keay, the surge in testosterone just before ovulation helps mature the egg to be ovulated.

"This is why some women with polycystic ovary syndrome (PCOS) [struggle with fertility]. High testosterone messes up ovulation, it stays high all the time and doesn't go up and down. Many women with PCOS still produce oestrogen, but because the testosterone is fixed, it will not allow ovulation to happen."

I'd assumed PCOS involved cysts, but this is only a small part of the picture. PCOS occurs when your ovaries produce too many androgens, male sex hormones, which disrupt the hormonal balance required for a healthy menstrual cycle and can lead to some combination of irregular periods, excess facial and/or body hair, weight gain, hair loss or thinning, insulin resistance (increasing your risk of type 2 diabetes) and difficulties in conceiving. You're born with it, although symptoms generally only start showing themselves in puberty, and for some women, not until their 20s. There's no definitive cure – but there are treatment options. Diet and exercise can help with the insulin resistance significantly, and medication can help ovaries to release eggs. The NHS website offers advice and support, so does Verity, the UK PCOS charity.

But if you don't have PCOS, if your oestrogen and testosterone are surging at ovulation in precisely the way they're supposed to, "it's a double whammy," according to Maisie Hill. "They're like a power couple."

A power couple that wants nothing more than for you to go out into the world and have unfettered sex in the name of getting pregnant. Like Jane Austen, but more lust-addled. Oooh! Like Bridgerton!

"Oestrogen is making you more positive – more energised – in that first phase of your cycle, when you're increasingly fertile. So whether you want to conceive or not, your body, your hormones, are driving you towards mating behaviour."

"The increase in energy – we're more out in the world, going out, curious, interested, flirty. 'Oh! Who can I mate with?' That's what the body's trying to do. And then testosterone is there, encouraging us to take risks: 'Look at *that* guy! Look at *that* one!' [Pushing us] to engage in that slightly riskier behaviour that is more likely to result in having sex and conceiving."

As Hill says this, as she speaks these words, I feel that visceral jolt of recognition you get when the facts behind this thing you instinctively understood, just knew – in your bones, in your cells, in the through-line of your female ancestors, in every coded conversation you've ever had with female friends – to be true, are laid out before you, in pretty non-negotiable biological terms. So much falls into place, all at once: years of behaviour, hundreds of mistakes, tens of shags I could definitely have done without. Texts sent, completely against my better judgement, numbers exchanged with blatant wrong 'uns, relapses into relationships I'd fought hard to leave just weeks before… I see it all, suddenly, so clearly, as having been nudged along by those hormonal surges. I would dearly love to see the receipts on past behaviour, how certain acts, certain un-take-back-able conversations intersect with my stage in any given menstrual cycle. How much grief, hilarity, awkwardness, inadvisable sh*t, could I have avoided, had I had a glimmer of awareness that I was probs not acting with my own best interests at heart, but at the behest of my surging oestrogen and testosterone? How different would my life look now, if I'd been in possession of all the hormonal facts?

Blimey.

Ah, but never mind: it's done now, it's over, the aftermaths have been absorbed, the sketchier interludes have run their course. I should move on.

Maisie Hill has.

"Immediately after ovulation, you go from feeling capable, confident, loving what you look like in the mirror, feeling really good about yourself, like you can do anything, to: 'Oh my God, why did I say that I can do that thing? Who am I to do that?' There can be that really stark difference."

Oh bloody hell, yes! I've had that, too!

"And that's because, hormonally, there's been that peak, and now it's coming down again."

Oestrogen and testosterone are dwindling suddenly, Progesterone is in charge?

"Think about it like a rollercoaster. Where you're getting going, then you're at the top, then you come down. There's a gradual second wave [of oestrogen] that happens post ovulation. It's not as steep or as sudden as in the first half…"

Or as fun?

"Ha. No. So there's a period of time where we're waiting for hormones to pick up again." This, according to Dr Nicky Keay's hormone graph, is around Day 17 of a 28-day cycle, when everything has bottomed out, apart from progesterone, which is on a slow rise, and before Days 19, 20, 21, when oestrogen increases again. "That's so important for people to know, because, if you don't, you end up questioning yourself. 'How come one week I can feel like this, and the next, I feel like this?'"

YES! I've had times when, say, I've written an article, and it's lairy and confident and provocative and bold, because that's how *I* was at the point of writing, but, by the time it came out, a week, maybe even just *days* later, I felt timid and terrified, amazed I ever had the gall, the chutzpah, to write that *thing*, not to mention quite incapable of handling any backlash from irate readers. And I never understood why, or which version of me was the true one, the real me. Am I lairy Polly or timid Polly?

"It's just your hormones! Give yourself a couple of days, take it easy on yourself, let things get going again."

Then what?

"Well, if the first half of the cycle is about getting you out there, getting you to have sex and procreate, the second half is more about keeping you safe in case you have [conceived]." So progesterone's dominance makes us more risk averse and insecure? That sudden lack of confidence is about keeping us and, specifically any potential pregnancy, very safe, at home, out of harm's way?

"Inclined to stay in, yeah. Or, if you are going out, people often talk about feeling more… specific, about who they want to be with. A bit more particular. *Choosy.* It's as if, the first half of our cycle, we've got rose-tinted glasses on."

Oestrogen-tinted glasses!

"Right. Because oestrogen wants you to get out there and have sex. Oestrogen doesn't want you focussed on the pile of dirty dishes your partner has left. Because then, you're not going to want to have sex with them. Whereas the second half of the cycle, we've got progesterone ruling, the rose-tinted glasses are off… We see the details that bother us. The ones we were able to gloss over in the first half of the cycle."

We become more critical of our partners – but also of ourselves?

"Definitely. And that's where the inner criticism and outer criticism come in and can be really debilitating for some people. Then, around the 21-day mark, that's when we get a peak in progesterone. Progesterone, for a lot of people – not everyone, but a lot – is very soothing on the nervous system. Progesterone helps us to sleep. So this is a really great phase to capitalise on sleep… rather than going out and staying out late."

In the couple of days before your period, when pretty much all your hormones have dipped really low, you can experience interrupted sleep, even full-on insomnia. This is thought to be a consequence of low oestrogen causing a rise in your body temperature, which can wake you up in the middle of the night, then prevent you dropping off again.

There's considerable evidence that women suffer more injuries in this luteal phase of our menstrual cycles, that we're more physically awkward, and that this can impact us significantly. I'll get to that – I've got a high-flying physio, and Dr Keay and all the work she's done with ballet dancers, all over it.

But I had wondered if we're also negatively affected *cognitively* in this phase. I've certainly felt less sharp, less on it, intellectually speaking, during and around my period. Is that due to the general lack of confidence Hill thinks is associated with my hormones trying to keep me and my notional pregnancy at home, away from danger? Or are we actually less sharp, less smart, more limited, more – y'know – *thick* in the latter stages of our menstrual cycle?

Absolutely not, according to Dr Sarah McKay, my New Zealander neuroscientist.

"I looked at studies of cognition," Dr McKay tells me. "The brain's cool because it can adapt across the menstrual cycle cognitively. We don't really see, at different points in the menstrual cycle, enormous shifts in our ability to cognitively perform, which is good. Imagine if we did. Oh, 'You're a bit useless at this time of the month but you're better at the other...'"

I can imagine how that might be used against us in a massive way, used to inhibit women's progression up the political ranks, or, to gaining their pilot's licence, or really anything powerful, well paid, well respected at all.

"Right."

PMS: PRE-MENSTRUAL SYNDROME

What about PMS? I ask both Dr McKay and Maisie Hill. It's caused by us having very low hormone levels, I can see that: but why does that make us so *angry*? Is it purely that the oestrogen goggles have come off, the world looks kinda foul without them and that just... *pisses us off*? Makes us feel cheated, short-changed, put-upon?

Hill thinks so.

"My thought on this is, we do the bulk of unpaid labour and emotional labour in society. When we have oestrogen dominating the scene, and it's all about us being attracted to someone, wanting to have sex with them, flirting... I've heard it called 'the accommodating hormone'. Wanda Sykes, the comedian, has this amazing bit in her stand-up which I love, where she talks about how, when you're in the supermarket, and someone bumps into you, *you* apologise... She's like: 'That's oestrogen.'"

So oestrogen keeps us nice, mostly, but...

"The anger is always there."

Oestrogen masks it?

"Totally. And then in that second half of the cycle, when we have a different hormonal landscape, whether it be low, whether progesterone is up, I think it just reveals what is there all the time. My take on it is: our hormones help us access that anger. But it's always there."

Dr Sarah McKay has strong scientific reasons to think PMS is profoundly influenced by our circumstances. She explored the idea in her book, *The Woman's Brain Book* (2018), and discovered that rates of PMS vary between 10% and 90% of women in a population, depending on whom you ask and where they live. In France, for example, around 10% of women say they have PMS, while in Iran, 90% of women claim to. As Dr McKay points out, if this were representative of a purely biological phenomenon, those figures couldn't exist; you can't possibly have a scenario in which almost everyone, yet at the same time, hardly anyone, suffers from PMS. Other studies, in which women were asked to rate their changing emotions across the course month without raising the issue of PMS, specifically found there really wasn't a big variation in the way women felt globally, over the course of their menstrual cycle. Dr McKay describes a paper that crunched the data on "hundreds and hundreds of women, hundreds and hundreds of cycles" and concluded that France's 10% of women with mood strongly influenced by PMS is globally representative. What, then, is happening in Iran? The researchers believe that 90% of women are actually talking about mood influenced by overall well-being – rather than mood influenced by hormones (or lack of). She thinks these women are dealing with stress and a lack of social support.

"There's an awful lot of data out there showing that things like

PMS are influenced by gendered experiences," she tells me. "In countries where there's big, gendered inequality, women are more likely to say they have PMS, because it's like they've actually got permission, at a certain point in the month, to be sh*tty with men. Whereas in countries where there's more gender equity, women have less PMS, because you can kind of be pissed off at any time of the month."

But for some, PMS is more than just feeling irritable or a bit pissed off. Much more. Premenstrual Dysphoric Disorder (PDD) is a severe, often under-recognised form of PMS. It can cause intense mood swings, anxiety, and depression that can really disrupt daily life. It usually kicks in during the two weeks before menstruation and can be managed with lifestyle changes or the help of a healthcare professional.

THE MENSTRUAL CYCLE AND MENTAL HEALTH

As she and I discuss the menstrual cycle from the neuroscientist's perspective, Dr McKay segues gently, but inevitably, into the territory of my recurring fears around whether having a female body negatively impacts mental health. She says that a girl who goes through puberty much earlier than her friendship group, but at a point which is still considered healthy, will be far more vulnerable to mood disorders than girls who get their periods at the same age as their friendship group, or slightly later. This seems to indicate that it's not the hormones per se, but rather the girl changing, her social context and her perception of herself and her friends.

Can this be applied to women and mental health in general? It is about our hormones – but it's also not about out hormones? Or not *only* about our hormones?

"Yeah. We've got our top-down propensities for rumination and internalising when we're experiencing stress in our lives, whereas men are more likely to externalise… we see biological sex playing a role. But we've also got gender playing a role. Maybe you're a teenager, you've gone on the pill, the pill is associated with slightly increased rates of depression [in teenage girls]… But that might be because you're a 14-year-old and you've gone on the pill because you're having a sexual relationship, and you can't cope. Was it the pill? Or was it the fact that you were in a sexual relationship when you were 14? I think we need to look at the biology and the sociology and the psychology, which all add up to there being this slight deviation. There was a paper published recently that looked at brains – there are really cool new ways of studying them. We've got these big bio-banks, huge data banks! Thousands of labs around the world have put all their brain-imaging data together. We can pool all the data. Power in numbers. We can use machine learning and AI to analyse the data; it doesn't have to be a little scientist with their spreadsheet in the lab any more, looking at 12 people's brain scans. We can look at 10,000 people at once! So they've looked at gender equality. All these countries from around the world, and you can rank them by how equal their genders are. Countries where there's really big gender inequality, where women are oppressed… we see *deficits* in brain structure, in the women compared to the men."

I find this study. It was published in 2023,[13] the lead author on

---

13 Country-level gender inequality is associated with structural differences in the brains of women and men, *Psychological and Cognitive Sciences*, 2023 – https://doi.org/10.1073/pnas.2218782120

it is Dr Nicolas Crossley, visiting professor in the Department of Psychiatry at the University of Oxford, and associate professor in the Pontificia Universidad Católica in Chile. Having looked at 7800 MRI brain scans of people from 29 different countries, the study concluded: "In countries where there was greater gender inequality, the cortical thickness of the right hemisphere of women's brains was thinner than men's. In more gender-equal countries there was no significant difference. The areas of the brain affected were those particularly associated with stress and emotions."

"These changes were particularly located in brain regions involved in control of emotions and that are also affected in stress-related disorders such as depression and post-traumatic stress disorder," Dr Crossley explained. "We therefore think that what we are seeing is the effect of chronic stress in women's brains in gender-unequal environments. Stress affects neurons' connections, which we would then see as thinning of the grey matter cortex in MRI studies. However, other mechanisms could also be involved, such as the effect of reduced opportunities, including education, in women's brains, leading to lower development of connections."

Or, if you'd rather: inequality screws lady brains right up.

PERFORMANCE AND THE MENSTRUAL CYCLE

In late 2019, the sports brand Nike was in the process of developing a training app. Megan Jones, a keen netball player, was part of the advertising company that was working with Nike on it. As the project began, Jones tore her ACL while playing netball. ACLs are anterior cruciate ligaments; they rest in the centre of the knee, serving a desperately important stabilising function in that delicate, crucial joint. They're becoming increasingly famous with particular reference to women's football and the issues they keep causing top-level players. At the time Jones hurt her ACL, she was playing a pre-season game. It was horrendous, she says, "the most painful thing". She fell to the ground. "One of my team-mates, a friend who's a surgeon, said: 'You went deadly silent. Medical training, you always worry about the silent ones. If people make noise, they're fine.'"

Another friend introduced her to Tom Bradley, founder and lead physiotherapist of Warrior Rehab, a man with 25 years' experience working with both professional athletes, and the rest of us. They worked on her injury through the course of 2020 – Bradley would introduce her to a surgeon – and he even "fought the case on my medical insurance for me, he was a legend." When the initial waves of abject pain subsided, a couple of physio sessions or so in, Megan Jones asked him: "Why have I done this?" In response, Bradley pointed her towards the increasing evidence showing how menstrual cycles influence women's bodies from a performance perspective. Over a couple of years proceeding Megan Jones's injury, Bradley, along with a small but deeply significant group of physios and doctors, had become increasingly interested in how the menstrual cycle affects women's physicality; how the luteal phase in particular, that last half of the cycle, seemed to coincide with a significantly increased tendency towards injury.

Jones – who'd just read Caroline Criado Perez's 2019 book *Invisible Women*, which looks at the absence of available data on women's bodies and how that negatively impacts us in every situation from transport to politics to: yup, medicine! – found this fascinating.

The advertising agency with which she was working at that time as a strategist had been briefed by Nike to try to improve the extent to which its existing training app engaged with women – "because it was low". Women would typically start using it, then drop out. Nike wondered how it might keep them there, keep them engaged. Jones – known by the agency to be of a sporty inclination – got called into a brainstorming meeting, to see if she could offer inspiration.

"This chat was right after one of my physio sessions. I said: 'I've just heard this around periods, and I think it might be fascinating to look into it.' Gave them some insights, you know: 'Women are more likely to get this injury at this point in their cycle…'"

This conversation prompted Nike to hire Dr Stacy Sims, author of *ROAR* (the 2016 book about the differences between male and female athletes) and the 2019 Ted "Talk Women Are Not Small Men", who has devoted her entire career to researching the impact of hormones on women and training. "She's fascinating," says Megan Jones. "She talks about how even diet culture is subject to this bias. We're all told to do keto, but that's all based on research on men in their 50s and 60s who need to lose weight before heart surgery. Actually, women need more carbohydrates, and at different points in our cycle, we need to eat different things."

In 2022, as a direct consequence of Megan Jones's sessions with Tom Bradley, and in association with Dr Stacy Sims, Nike launched NikeSync, an app-based training programme designed to help women work with their hormones, rather than against them; to focus (for example) on strength and cardio when our hormones are supporting us, and mobility and good form when they leave us fatigued, more vulnerable to injuries and so on.

If this all sounds a bit far-fetched to you, a bit faddy and foolish, then please know that:

a) Chelsea Women's team has been fully committed to this training approach since around 2019 when it first started to track its players' cycles, and vary their training in step with it, and that team is "the most successful in Women's Super League history;"[14] and

b) as Dr Nicky Keay points out: "75% of doping infringements are hormone-related. The athletes know it, unscrupulous doctors and trainers and whatever know it: hormones are key to performance." If we understand and accept that artificial hormones dramatically affect performance – and clearly, we do; doping authorities *certainly* do – then it certainly follows that natural hormonal fluctuations can influence performance, too, sometimes negatively.

I meet Tom Bradley to find out more. It's not my first meeting with Bradley, by any means. If Megan Jones did all of 2020 with him, I did late 2020 into early 2021. I injured a disc in my lower thoracic spine while Zoom training like a mad woman – every day, sometimes more – to alleviate the boredom and fear of Covid's lockdowns. Being that injured was *awful*. I couldn't walk for more than 10 minutes at a time for two months after the injury. I was in constant, nagging pain, which stopped me sleeping. My mood was low, which had nothing to do with my menstrual cycle, and everything to do with me not being able to

---

14 Chelsea leading the charge in women's football on and off the pitch, 2025 – https://theprideoflondon.com/chelsea-leading-the-charge-in-women-s-football-on-and-off-the-pitch-01jkz1pjphdw

amp up my endorphins with physical exercise. I spent six months getting back to full spine health, much of which was overseen by Bradley, to whom I owe my now magnificently restored spine mobility, and also, my mind. As in the case of Megan Jones, Bradley was the first person with whom I ever had a conversation about the impact of the menstrual cycle on women in terms of performance and injury.

Tom Bradley has been working as a physio for 25 years; he began his career in the NHS before working with male rugby and football players, then moving on to the tennis circuit, working with both male and female players, and finally opening his own private practice, "working with normal humans", in 2018. As a passionate and curious therapist, he started noticing patterns in how women sustained injuries, how they were different from men and their injuries. He began wondering how we might better protect our bodies against injury, or heal them more efficiently, should we pick one up.

We begin by talking about the paucity of studies on female athletes, compared to male. Because there is really very little. As Dr Paulina Kloskowska, lecturer in physiotherapy at King's College London, noted in her 2023 paper: "Female athletes are underrepresented in all areas of medical research, particularly sports research. There is little female-specific data that would inform the training, rehab, prehab and exercise protocols for women athletes – and all guidelines are currently based on data based on male athletes."[15]

---

15 The need for further research into female athletes in sports research, 2023 – https://www.kcl.ac.uk/female-athletes-sports-research#:~:text=Female%20athletes%20are%20underrepresented%20in,data%20based%20on%20male%20athletes

Men's sports, Bradley points out, were professional long before women's sports, which accounts for it, but it's frustrating and, in some situations, terribly misleading. "In things like football and rugby, all the [research into] conditioning, injury prevention, dietetics, *everything* has been cut and pasted from men's sport into female sport."

This is a problem because, as Dr Stacy Sims puts it in the title of her course on women's physiology: "Women are not small men." You cannot simply shrink the stats to account for differences in body size and assume they'll apply. For a whole range of reasons – into which, we're about to delve – they just won't.

OK, so wild guess *but* (I say to Tom Bradley), if there's very little medical research into female athletes and how their biology impacts their performance, there's going to be less still on women who aren't athletes?

"Yes."

But would it be reasonable to take the observations of the small amount of work that has been done on female athletes, then apply it to the rest of us?

"I think so."

Bradley himself has the benefit of years of experience working with non-professional athletes, observing the way our bodies work – and stop working when injured.

There are, he says, three major forces at play on the female body, from a physiotherapeutic perspective, the menstrual cycle, perimenopause and menopause.

Women exercising through their 30s and 40s, he continues, often don't understand, or aren't even aware, how their menstrual cycle affects the way they train, how it will fluctuate from month

to month, how it fluctuates yet more as they move towards perimenopause – and how those fluctuations can lead to issues. "It's
like a huge moving feast of elements, and nobody's really got an
idea of what's normal, how you should train, and how you should
recover."

All of which impacts performance?

"Yes."

In younger women, women in their 20s and early 30s – "post-
school, pre-perimenopause women" – a group most likely to be
still involved in team sports like netball – there are, Bradley says,
higher incidences of injuries, like the ACL tear Megan Jones
suffered, than there are in men. (Coincidentally, I met up with
Bradley in the summer of 2023, two days after the FIFA
Women's World Cup ended – a tournament hit hard by ACL
injuries; many of the world's best players were out of the competition on account of them, England superstars Beth Mead and
Leah Williamson among them.)

OK – so why? Why might this subset of women be injuring
themselves in this particular way?

"The research points to how, in certain phases of the menstrual
cycle – the late follicular into luteal – there are changes in core
body temperature."

It rises, right? Which interrupts your sleep, which makes you
more tired and less coordinated, I say (remembering the nail
technician who once, while giving me a pedicure, asked if I had
my period. "Yes!" I said, amazed and bemused, because how
could she possibly know that, just by looking at my feet? She
explained she'd noticed a couple of newish bruises on my ankles,
which suggested I'd just been through a phase of clumsiness,
which tended to coincide with the 48 hours right before a period

starts – which made me think she was basically the Sherlock Holmes of period deduction. Seriously, this is the basis for a massive plot twist in a legal drama, no?)

"Yes," says Bradley, "but also, when your oestrogen and progesterone are swapping dominance, you begin to have issues with fatigue, coordination and muscular strength. Oestrogen has an effect on your mitochondria."

Mitochondria, he explains, are like a sort of factory within each of your muscle cells, whose purpose is to produce energy. They're influenced by fluctuations in hormones, because they too have oestrogen receptors, which means that at certain points in the menstrual cycle, your body is less efficient at a cellular level, less good at breaking down and producing the chemicals required to form muscle contractions – so you can't move as efficiently, or as quickly; and you're less strong.

Furthermore, you're more tired, because your sleep has been disrupted by a rise in your core body temperature, due to the effects of increased progesterone levels. This means that if you're trying to play a multi-directional sport like netball or football, you are more likely to sustain something like an ACL injury. Your proprioception – your sense of where you are physically in space, where different parts of your body are, relative to each other, and how much force is required to move them for a desired result – is compromised.

And – to bring this out of the athletic zone and into real life briefly – if you're not playing netball, but say, running for a bus dodging traffic, carrying too many bags which are unevenly distributed across your body and, I dunno, trying to control a slightly wayward dog on a lead, while in your luteal phase… that could cause some trouble too?

"You're going to catch fewer buses in that particular week, yes." In addition to which, he points out, your body will often swell slightly, particularly around the abdomen and breasts, which changes the way it interacts with other parts of itself. It's suddenly, temporarily heavier and more cumbersome in some places than it was two days ago.

Plus: "If you're sore and uncomfortable, you're not going to move as athletically. And *then*, you have to think about where your ovaries and uterus are. If they're sore [which they probably are, because of that inflammation controlled by the prostaglandins, which trigger your period], the fascial connections – the connective tissue that surrounds and links muscles, ligaments, tendons, and organs – can create tension that extends into your hip flexors and back into your lumbar spine [the lower end of your spinal column]. An increase in body temperature and inflammation, and you're moving into a higher index risk of developing back pain. Can you believe I'm man-splaining periods to you?"

You're not man-splaining, so much as physio-splaining: it's really not a problem when a man with superior medical knowledge tells me something I didn't already know, though how did I not know this? *How?*

Bradley emphasises how important it is to track data such as heart rate variability and sleep quality. If male athletes were showing the sort of fluctuations that are routine in women because of the menstrual cycle, their training would be adapted to protect them from possible injury. However, female athletes are going through that, every month, without anyone issuing equivalent warnings or recommending equivalent precautions.

I got into fitness at 40, most unexpectedly. I'd spent my adult life to that point dodging it, then sort of stumbled over the whole shebang, discovered I adored it and really welcomed the impact it made on my body, how strong I suddenly felt. But as my experience of fitness progressed, as I became increasingly aware of my body and its potential, I also started noticing all the times it seemed to fail me, slightly. All the times I felt mysteriously less good on the Pilates mat than I had the session before, less strong, less stable, less able to get up into a bridge or sustain a plank; how I faltered in my weekly boxing class, tired more quickly, punched the bag less accurately; all the moments I frustrated myself by being not as good, as strong, as powerful as I had, the week before. And all the ways I blamed myself when I slipped off a pavement curb, or flipped my ankle while turning round because someone had called my name; all the times I called myself a "stupid cow", assumed I was being lazy, not working hard enough, or just abstractly crap – when in fact, my hormones were dipping, there was nothing I could have done about it, other than dial it down a little, stay in bed a little longer, focus on recovery, give myself a break.

It should be said that the menstrual cycle is not the only factor that makes women's bodies more vulnerable to injury than men's. There are musculoskeletal realities, the impact of our breasts and our broader hips on our movement, for example; there are societal factors, historically different expectations around boys and girls, whom sport was for, whom it suits – a 2022 study published by Sports England suggested that 64% of girls have dropped out of sport by the age of 16–17.[16] Then come ideas around femininity, how that might discourage us from moving freely and acquiring visible muscle mass. There's the gender gap in exercise, which sees significantly fewer women than men exercising, and citing lack of time, money and low self-confidence as reasons for giving up on fitness or not attempting it in the first place.[17]

There's also the not unimportant fact that our very feet are formed differently: for years, female footballers had been forcing themselves into boots designed for male feet. They had been so used, as women, to the idea that shoes just hurt, they'd literally run with it. More on this below.

But for now, and with specific reference to the menstrual cycle: what do women do? I ask Tom Bradley. Give up? Play less demanding sport?

"No! You have to track your menstrual cycle. You have to know yourself. If you think about how something this fundamental, the physical process of menstruation, the menstrual cycle, all of the changes, the fluctuations in hormones that are very important to how you feel, how you move, how you think, how you perform, how you feel emotionally and physically: if you are able to have the best possible understanding of that, as you move through the course of the month, you can then test things around it. Sleep strategies. Dietary strategies. Exercise strategies."

Your exercise regime should align with your cycle – ease off the high-intensity interval training when your hormonally

---

16 We need to keep pushing, *Sport England*, 2022 – https://www.sportengland.org/blogs/we-need-keep-pushing

17 Closing the gender gap, *ASICS*, 2023 – https://cms-static.asics.com/media-libraries/104783/file.pdf

overloaded system needs a break, and switch to Pilates, or even moderate weights instead. When you're feeling back at full power, you can ramp up it again. Although we currently lack research to fully confirm a need to train in line with different menstrual cycle stages, the basic rule – that your body is constantly giving you clues about what it needs on any given day and that you should listen to it – always applies. If you haven't slept well, if you're feeling low on energy – train, or rest, in accordance.

ACLS – ANTERIOR CRUCIATE LIGAMENTS

This is a diversion from my pure consideration of the menstrual cycle but – as is clear from my conversation with Tom Bradley – it's in no sense unrelated, and it's a truly necessary one. I know this because, nine times out of ten, when I tell someone I'm working on a book about women's bodies, they say: "Are you going to do ACLs?" Awareness of how this is an injury towards which women are especially inclined peaked in the summer of 2023, when the FIFA Women's World Cup was *devastated* by them, with vast swathes of popular players ruled out, on account of them, and speculation on why they were happening began to run rife.

The cursed female ACL comes up pretty quickly when I meet Anna Deignan, a former elite footballer, to talk about her perspective on women's bodies. We start our conversation by talking about feet. I'd just learned, from a friend who also works in professional football, that until relatively recently, everyone had assumed women's feet were identical to men's feet, if (generally) smaller. As a consequence, football boots had just been scaled down for female players – only, as it turns out, our feet are actually rather differently formed altogether, so ramming them into boots designed for men, then shrunk, does not cut it.

"Oh God! *Polly*! This drove me *mad* throughout my entire playing career! It's something about women having a narrower Achilles-to-heel ratio? There are still, I think, only a few boot manufacturers who are making boots for women. We are differently shaped! We really are. Plus, I'm convinced our foot shape changes as we get older. I noticed my foot has broadened... I think I went up a size in boot, even though I am the same physical build, and I'm convinced that's a hormonal thing. I think it happens after you give birth."

Deignan played competitively for Arsenal and QPR, before retiring and moving into government, where she was head of sport in the Department of Digital, Culture, Media and Sport. "Now, I'm at the Premier League, among other things working with the Football Association, women's pro game and others to take women's football to the next level." Deignan has played football "since the age of four. Back in the dark ages when there were no girls' teams, I had to go with the boys' teams. To see the trajectory the women's game is on is so exciting for me." She's now in her mid-40s. She had to stop playing football very recently following the diagnosis of a heart problem, so she's been hitting the gym instead ("It's not about vanity, it's about the future and bone health. Though granted, it's nice that I feel quite buff,"); but her playing years were intense. "I had lots of injuries along the way, so I was acutely aware of my physicality." Her style of play was very combative, very physical, she tells me. She broke her nose three times, for example, regularly had stitches in her face. "But... I found it liberating. I was very fair, very clean, but it mattered to me that, as women competing in sport, we are physical beasts – we want to win, and it's fine to bring that aggression. And I miss it. Maybe aggression isn't the word?"

Oh, I think it is, I say. I started boxing training a few years ago, as part of an all-women's boxing group, and I was amazed and delighted by how aggressive I can be when I'm allowed, how exciting it is to be around other women, all of whom are honouring and releasing their own aggression. I think aggression is *exactly* the word!

"Yes! I think you're right!" says Deignan.

I ask her if she thinks the level of physicality experienced at the top level of sport affects female bodies differently. She pauses, then says she thinks it does. She's had nine surgeries on her knee. "I did the legendary ACL injury, first in one knee, when I was about 19, at Arsenal, then I did the other ACL about five years later, when I was at QPR." From that unfortunate starting point, she'd go on to have multiple other surgeries. This is, she thinks, at least partly about the shape of her body. "Although I'm certainly androgynous presenting, my physique is very classically female. I have big boobs and broad hips." Those hips, she notes, are great for childbearing, but are potentially something of which to be mindful, when playing top-level sport. She is convinced, from all the conversations she's had with orthopaedic surgeons and physios over the years, that there is something about hip–knee ratio and alignment that contributes to injury rates. The issue with ACLs in particular, she says, is that football involves a lot of "cutting" – the rapid stopping and changing of direction – which means as a player, you're repeatedly putting all your weight onto one knee in one position, then suddenly, dramatically, shifting it.

A paper published in June 2023 by the British Orthopaedic

Association (BOA),[18] authored by Morgan Bailey, consultant trauma and orthopaedic surgeon based at University Hospital Southampton and Portsmouth University Hospital, and Nathaneal Ahearn, consultant trauma and orthopaedic surgeon for Torbay and South Devon Hospitals, confirms Deignan's instinct – cutting is a significant contributing factor in creating ACL injuries in women. It found that:

Biologically female athletes had 3–6 times higher risk of ACL injury than males, and that this was due to a multitude of reasons. One of these is the menstrual cycle.

"There is no doubt that hormonal influences on ligament laxity… put the average biologically female player on the back foot"; in addition to which, the paper cited a higher likelihood of valgus lower-limb alignment in women, the medical term for what is rather rudely but much more widely known as knock knee, a condition more common in women. "In women's football the majority (88%) of injuries are non-contact and are associated in two-thirds of cases with defensive pressing. It is a horizontal movement (rapid deceleration)… combined with single-leg loading and a change of direction [i.e. cutting] that is the mechanism of ACL injury." The BOA report also referenced the negative influence of football's "gendered environment", specifically poor-quality pitches, less-qualified coaches and "the fact that women's football boots are smaller versions of those

---

18　How to tackle the increased rate of ACL injuries in women's football, *BOA*, 2023 – https://www.boa.ac.uk/resource/how-to-tackle-the-increased-rate-of-acl-injuries-in-women-s-football.html

designed for men, rather than women specific."

"The male body just can absorb more strain and impact than ours," Deignan thinks. "In the gym, I need an objective, and my objective is to be able to do more pull-ups. I don't know if you can." I can't. "It's quite unusual for women to be able to do them. What really annoys me, the men around me, in the office even, are not even half fit, but they have 40% greater upper-body strength, just naturally. I hate to say it, because I think women are made of steel and I love us to bits, but that resilience to blows [is not as great]. In my experience, the healing time is a little bit longer for women."

I find research which suggests that, yup, women's lower muscle mass means they do recover from strains and sprains more slowly than men. I also find evidence that we sustain concussion more easily, but recover more rapidly.

"Maybe some of this is testosterone," Deignan goes on, "which enables men to play on through pain more." A 2015 study found that testosterone was an effective way to treat fibromyalgia, the chronic pain condition that mainly affects women.[19] "That said, whenever I've had, or witnessed, a serious injury on a woman, she doesn't complain, she just sucks it up, while the men tend to be in a bit of a state." She thinks there are two things at play: men's physical strength, which makes them better able to move their body through the planes of motion, and their actual anatomy. "I'm not an anatomy expert, but when you look at the male body, and it's that sort of straight line, shoulders, then narrow

---

19 A novel use for testosterone to treat central sensitization of chronic pain in fibromyalgia patients, *International Immunopharmacology*, 2015 – https://doi.org/10.1016/j.intimp.2015.05.020

hips and straight down to the ankles, there's just less room for that excess of motion..."

Which results in less injury?

"Yeah. So when I watch a male elite player, versus a female elite player, at equivalent levels, change direction after a sprint, if they suddenly have to cut, I've noticed a small but noticeable lag in the turning time of women, and I think that's to do with where our centre of gravity is. We have more momentum, [so changing] direction, and turning back, is trickier."

Tom Bradley confirms that most of the ACL injuries he sees in women are a consequence of cutting.

Is this, I ask, perhaps about football itself? Is it a game designed around men's bodies, which needs to be reconfigured for women's bodies – like the boots? I understand some people are already actively arguing for the reduction of the size of the pitch and the goals specifically for the women's game. The mighty Emma Hayes, who took Chelsea's women's teams to such heights, is among them; she insists this isn't remotely sexist. "Try to set emotion aside and consider some facts," she wrote in *The Times*, in 2019, "such as the average height of a goalkeeper in men's football being at least six foot one inch – latest figures put it as high as six foot three inches in the Premier League – with goal-keepers in the Women's Super League about five foot eight inches. That is a significant disparity, particularly when the dimensions of a full-size outdoor goal are eight foot high and 24 foot wide."

Bradley says maybe; but that the ACL injuries he treats most commonly come from skiing, which is a pretty gender-neutral activity, and netball, a sport we probably instinctively think is played primarily by women, in which cutting plays an even bigger part than in football. "Particularly when you're jumping onto one leg and pivoting at the same time," he says. The Q-angle, the quadriceps angle, which we first encountered in the chapter on puberty, also has a part to play in these injuries.

"But I also think, if we take an honest look at the differences between men and women, men generate more muscular power," Bradley tells me. This isn't sexism either. It's just true. Men have a greater cross-sectional area of muscle, which makes them stronger, by around 20% as a ballpark, Bradley tells me. This inherent strength gives them an advantage in terms of injury in general, and ACLs specifically.

All of which means, says Anna Deignan, that women must focus on developing strength, above all. To do that, we need to strength-train hard – and completely disregard the cultural imperative towards spindly, slender, less-strong ideas of femininity.

"All of this stuff that's peddled," she goes on, "that women's muscles need to be not visible, just lithe and lean… it's rubbish. And it's discouraging women from connecting with that physical strength."

WOMEN, ADDICTION, THE MENSTRUAL CYCLE (AND BEYOND)

I don't know about you, but I have always had a nagging sense that intoxicants hit the ladies harder. That booze, fags and illegals might hurt us more than they hurt men. I rail against it, too, because it seems so damned sexist – grist to the narrative that women should be sensible and mild and keep themselves neat and tidy and sane and sober, because we're basically society's grown-ups, or some such restrictive nonsense. Drinking and smoking and silliness and wildness? That's men's business! Being off your tits in the club? Men's business! And if women get drunk, it's basically our fault if we get raped. And if women get spiked, it's basically our fault for even being out in the first place, loitering in bars, when we should just be at home, sipping our water and eating our greens, keeping ourselves safe and sound and clean and serene in physical and emotional anticipation of our eventually achieving our One True Purpose: getting pregnant and having babies!

So reductive, no? So controlling!

And yet, I could not help but notice that I seemed to suffer more than my male friends, and my boyfriends, in the course of, and the wake of, a night out. That I'd get drunk quicker and more aggressively, have worse hangovers. Cigarettes – which I smoked sporadically and unconvincingly in my late teens and early 20s, 100% because I thought it made me look cool – could make me physically sick, actually puke, pretty regularly, while the men I knew? Never! And the drugs I (definitely never) took, (because they're illegal)? Could it really be that they made me feel more intensely, scarily, violently high, more quickly, then left me with rougher comedowns? Was that my imagination? My internalised misogyny, making me feel less able to keep up?

Or was it a consequence of something more fundamental in my female make-up?

Yeah. You guessed it. It's that last one.

"We know women drag in more toxins," says Dr Sharon Cox, a funny, dry, sweary, whip-smart academic who's biked in to meet me in my local caff. She's a principal research fellow in behavioural science and health at University College London and works within the Tobacco and Alcohol Research Group.

"My primary interest is the psychology of addictive behaviour. I've spent nigh on 20 years researching it."

And yes, she says, cigarettes and alcohol hurt us more than they hurt men.

Why?

"There are differences in the way we consume. There are differences in the way it's marketed. There are differences in the impact."

I ask her about the physiological differences; first, the biological ones.

"Alcohol and the effect on women's bodies: women do suffer more."

Why?

"We are more fatty than men, so the rate at which we metabolise alcohol is slower. If we drink the same as men, we will get more unwell. We also can, often do, end up with a lot more damage."

And that's because of fat?

"Yes. Naturally, we're fatter than men. I'm not saying we're fatter proportionally, just that we have [a higher percentage of] body fat so it's harder for alcohol to get out of our system."

So because it sits in our bodies for longer, which means we're exposed to it for longer, it does more harm?

"Yes. Also, when you're ovulating, your body will prioritise ovulation above metabolising alcohol, so we get pissed quicker when we're ovulating."

No. Friggin'. Way. That's one of those things I *kind* of knew…

"But you didn't know!"

Exactly! So, at the point of ovulation, our body is basically saying: "Get pregnant! All other physical processes can go to hell while you do that!"

"Yup… it's a complex process of breaking down alcohol in the gut, sending it to the liver, creating alcohol enzymes and getting rid of it through the kidneys, through sweat, breath and urine. If you're ovulating as well, your body prioritises that."

Dr Cox's work also shows it's harder for us to give up cigarettes when we're ovulating – again, because our body cares about nothing but conception, therefore, by definition, things like self-control and delayed gratification are not our strong suits. Why would they be? Self-control and delayed gratification tend to get in the way of our going out and having lots of sex, after all. We're also more likely to relapse into addictions while ovulating. This has been proven in women in the case of smoking; and according to a 2019 study published by the National Institute of Drug Abuse in the US, working in tandem with the University of Maryland, cocaine addiction might well be similarly impacted by ovulation. It discovered that female rats craved cocaine during periods of abstinence[20] much more strongly when they were ovulating than at any other point; also, that they were more likely to relapse than male rats. A 2021 study, again on rats, found that female rats have a greater response than male rats to stimulants like amphetamines and cocaine throughout their cycle, which, it concluded, was partly related to the presence of oestradiol. If the idea that women suffer greater cravings and relapse more regularly than men is contested in scientific

---

20 I'm assuming the scientists had artificially addicted the rats beforehand, not that they'd picked up expensive coke habits while loitering in the skirting boards of private members' clubs, though that presumably can and does happen.

and medical communities, which it is – only certain scientists believe that it is a factor – the idea we struggle harder with addiction at certain points in our menstrual cycle than at others is not disputed at all.

I ask Dr Cox if women get addicted more quickly than men, a theory I'd read in yet another study.

"Hmmmm. I think there's something about: our tolerance being lower? That we can handle less? That's different to addiction. We do see women consuming more alcohol than we used to."

Why?

"Tough times. Women have a lot to deal with. A lot to escape. And substances are a very reliable friend. If you can go to your shop, buy a bottle of wine, a packet of cigarettes, or go and see your dealer, pick up some coke, you know it's going to work. They're quick fixes."

This, Dr Cox says, is despite addiction being perceived as more abhorrent in women than men, which makes us less likely to seek help than men, more likely to hide our addictions.

"It always has been. Look at Hogarth's *Gin Lane*."

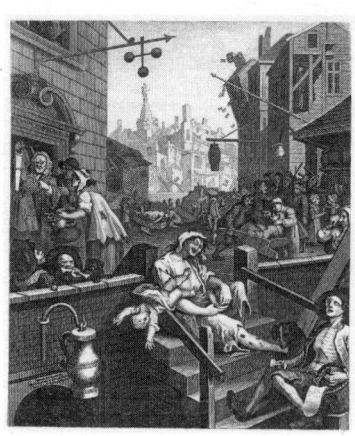

"The main character is a woman who's *dropping her baby*. It's seen as horrid, the worst thing you can do, and this is what she's allowing drink to do to her. 'Mother's Ruin' has come from that."

Because of all of this – or despite it, or both – Dr Cox believes addiction in women is actually more likely to have an emotional cause, a stress response, triggered by societal pressures, and expectations and ideas around achieving perfect motherhood, rather than a physical cause, a consequence of our bodies – our hormones, or our fat disposition – driving us towards it.

But physical factors are definitely at play, when we consider the interaction between the menstrual cycle and drugs.

Our relatively elevated oestrogen levels mean that we metabolise nicotine more quickly than men, which means we experience a more rapid and more intense experience of withdrawal, which is associated in turn with a lower success rate when attempting to quit cigarettes or nicotine.[21] This becomes worse yet, Dr Cox explains, when we're ovulating, or when we're pregnant, because we metabolise it much faster at these times. In addition, women have *huge* cravings when they're pregnant.

Why? Because it's physiologically harder to give up *anything* when you're pregnant or ovulating? Because your body is so focussed on that biological function, it can't really do anything else?

"Particularly nicotine. Very few women drink alcohol when they're pregnant. Very few." But 8.8% of British women were known to be smokers at the time of delivery, according to most

---

21 Nicotine chemistry, metabolism, kinetics and biomarkers, *Handb Exp Pharmacol*, 2009 – https://pmc.ncbi.nlm.nih.gov/articles/PMC2953858/

recent available figures[22] (which, as Dr Cox points out, won't be accurate: how many women wouldn't have admitted to smoking while pregnant, given the enormous stigma attached to it?) "Another reason women smoke when pregnant is that it's a sense of identity for them. They've given up their body, their time to this child, it's the only thing left." In addition to which: "Women who are pregnant, who smoke, are less likely to come to antenatal classes. There's this new [NHS] intervention, which is paying women to stay smoke-free." In April 2023, the British government announced that it would be offering incentives, in the form of vouchers, alongside behavioural support, to encourage pregnant smokers to stop. "The intervention is to help the child, because if your mother smokes, or your father, you're much more likely to take up smoking. So we want to protect that next generation. It's £2 a day. It's not a lot. But it's controversial, because [of the cultural expectation that] women should Just Give Up, for their baby. But women tell us they find it really hard. Or… this is really common: lots of women manage to give up smoking in pregnancy, but relapse post pregnancy. The longer you quit, the more likely you are to stay quit, but there's something in women post-partum, where they relapse. Nicotine is a fantastic suppressor of appetite." So because we're so desperate to lose baby weight, so convinced we must, by a fattist society that still, fundamentally, believes a woman's principal concern should be to be, and remain, thin and f*ckable – we pick the fags up again?

"Yeah. I mean, there's that desire to be desirable, that substances

---

22 Smoking in Pregnancy, *Nuffield Trust*, 2024 – https://www.nuffieldtrust.org.uk/resource/smoking-in-pregnancy

can help with – or at least we're told they can… Nicotine, vapes, cigarettes give you something to do with your hands so if you're hungry…"

You're distracted?

"Yup."

Dr Cox's work has led her to believe that women are operating at a disadvantage in the face of addiction, not just because of how our bodies process (or don't process) drugs, how our menstrual cycle can make us more vulnerable to addictive substances, how frenziedly we're trying to escape daily stressors, but also because of how aggressively addictive substances are marketed at us.

"The thing that women get, that men don't get, is: 'Take this substance, look desirable!' Oh, but: 'Don't take too much, because then you're undesirable!' Or as Gwyneth Paltrow said: 'I can only have one pint, because then I'm not attractive to my husband.'" (NB: I was not able to locate this quote from Gwyneth.)

"We've seen a huge increase in women being targeted with alcohol. Prosecco brunches? Gin o'clock? You'll see on Mother's Day, for example: 'Free Prosecco for Mum!' Or some shops might do offers where you'll get [deals on] alcohol for mum. Some of the biggest changes in the alcohol market are being tailored towards women. When women become more financially independent, they're seen as a new market. In Southeast Asia, for example, we are now seeing more women take up smoking. Men have always smoked in places like India. But some of the fastest-growing groups of smokers are middle-class women."

So in economies where women are acquiring money and independence and social capital for the first time – they're also being aggressively marketed at, for addiction?

"Yes."

I spend the next months noticing these "gags" everywhere I go; I eventually start screenshotting my favourites and sending them to Dr Cox, who, it turns out, collects them. I find workout vests which read "Prosecco and Pilates", baby-grows emblazoned with the words "I'm the reason Mummy needs wine". I find a newly sober lifestyle blogger talking about the targeting of mothers specifically with multiple messages about how fun and freeing and necessary it is to drink; such a weird twist on the Gin Lane, Mother's Ruin narrative, yet one which is also, somehow, connected to it surely?

This general widespread cultural assimilation of the idea that it's just super fun for women to drink started, Dr Cox tells me, as a concerted effort by manufacturers to make booze more female.

"Google 'Don't Pink My Drink,'" she suggests.

I do. I find a campaign by a substance-use research group at Glasgow Caledonian University, led by Professor Carol Emslie, which she kickstarted after she observed that, while men still drink more than women, that gap is narrowing, rapidly, and with dangerous consequences. "In the UK, alcohol-specific deaths in women have increased by 39% since 2001," she's reported. "We also know that alcohol is responsible for about 8% of breast cancers worldwide ... We've seen a move away from sexualising women to sell alcohol to men, towards alcohol brands trying to align their products with sophistication, women's empowerment and with female friendship," Professor Emslie adds. "This is really straight out of the tobacco industry playbook, with slogans such as 'You've come a long way, baby' in the 60s."

Meanwhile, Dr Sharon Cox tells me: "Women have always used substances. There's a woman called Marty Mann, she was one of the first spearheads of AA [Alcoholics Anonymous]. AA has always been attributed to two men" – Bill Wilson, known as Bill W., and Bob Smith, or Dr Bob – "but it was Marty Mann who was the first woman to go all the way through AA, to do the 12 steps."

Wikipedia's page on Mann begins:

Marty Mann
Margaret Marty Mann (October 15, 1904 – July 22, 1980) was an American writer who is considered by some to be the first woman to achieve long-term sobriety in Alcoholics Anonymous.

"This was in New York in the 40s and 50s," Dr Cox goes on. "She wrote books on it, and she'd go on the radio, but the thing about Marty was, she wasn't criticised, because she was middle class. She was a moneyed woman, she'd turn up at the interviews, well suited, well heeled. She was reputable. You couldn't have had a working-class woman from the Bronx talking like that." Dr Cox's greater point is: "Substance abuse happens in a gendered context, but also in a class context."

This, she thinks, is why addiction is much more evident in women lower down the socio-economic scale, with lives that involve far greater struggles – and many more reasons to look for escape – yet with far fewer means to relieve the stress of struggles by, say, checking into a spa, or going on a really lovely holiday. As a consequence, the idea that addiction is genetic, inherited, annoys Dr Cox.

"We talk about a genetic predisposition – but I fail to see how all these people with genetic vulnerabilities [always] come from poorer backgrounds, with terrible lives. I don't buy that.

"There are genetic vulnerabilities, which possibly are expressed maladaptively, in certain environments. So if someone's naturally a risk taker, in the right environment, with money and opportunity, they might... get into racing car driving. But if you're a young kid in Pollokshaws, Glasgow, and there are few opportunities, and people are giving out five-pound bags of heroin? That is your racing car."

Are women's hangovers really worse than men's? I ask Dr Cox.

"Yeah. Particularly if we're drinking while ovulating."

Because we're metabolising the booze badly?

"And because our blood sugar levels drop more rapidly, so we need more hydrating."

Studies demonstrate that, in the follicular stage, that first half of our cycle, rising oestrogen increases our sensitivity to insulin, which lowers blood sugar levels. Moreover, as we get older, we find it harder again to metabolise alcohol, so hangovers become worse. This is exacerbated during the menopause, when our oestrogen levels drop.

Dr Cox also tells me about a colleague, Dr Sally Adams, assistant professor at the University of Bath, whose research interests lie in "the cognitive and neurobiological mechanisms that underpin addictive behaviours," according to her LinkedIn. Dr Adams has found that, as women get older, they feel their hangovers are worse when they subjectively rate them. They also start to feel more guilty about drinking.

More guilty than when we were younger?

"And more guilty about drinking than men."

So our hangovers, or at least our perception of their severity, might be a form of self-punishment? We're sort of *making* ourselves feel worse? Or perhaps, experiencing our guilt as physical pain? Because we think we're too old to be behaving like this?

"Yes! And then, there's *another* twist to this, which is: women who've had children, regardless of their age, also report feeling more guilt and more pain when they're hungover.

"It's likely the feeling of guilt is intertwined with pain. 'I'm in pain because I feel ashamed, I feel ashamed because I'm in pain.'"

Later, I'll realise that what we're actually confronting here is indisputable evidence that alcohol is harder on women at all points of our lives. We get drunk more quickly when we're ovulating, our hangovers feel worse because our blood sugar level is more volatile then – but our hangovers are also worse later in our lives, because we feel guiltier then about drinking at all. Perimenopause and menopause make women yet less capable of metabolising alcohol because of falling oestrogen levels, but also because – according to Dr Fatima Khan, a menopause specialist based in Melbourne, Australia – levels of an enzyme in our liver, devoted to breaking alcohol down and ultimately eliminating it, dip, simply because of age.[23]

Dr Cox and I talk about nicotine patches, commonly used as a support to help people quit smoking, but which, I'd heard, might work less well for women.

"They can do."

Why?

---

23 How does alcohol affect menopause and perimenopause, *HCF*, 2023 – https://www.hcf.com.au/health-agenda/women/perimenopause-menopause/alcohol-and-menopause

"Metabolising, again. So what we would recommend, if you're ovulating, is using something like a slow-release patch that works in the background, then some fast release when you're on your cravings – something like a mouth spray. The whole goal is: don't worry about how much nicotine you're using in these forms, just don't smoke. So have a patch on, and if you're ovulating, or you're stressed – you're a woman and you've got things that will make you stressed in life, you have those moments where you think: 'F*ck it, I want a cigarette – don't. Just reach for the mouth spray. Reach for the vape. Don't worry about how much nicotine you're using. Just don't smoke.'"

This, I realise, is the major recurring theme in all the conversations I have, with all the experts, regarding the menstrual cycle and the ways it influences our physiology, behaviours and moods. Awareness of it, of what it means to all women hormonally, but also how that makes *you*, specifically, feel... That alone is a profoundly powerful thing. If you want to manage your mood, if you want to avoid injury, support your physical performance, if you want to avoid relapsing into an addiction, or calling an ex, or having daft sex... knowing where you are in your menstrual cycle and how that impacts you, in particular, is key – because we're all so incredibly individual, right? Not all of us will feel Beyoncé fire emoji when ovulating; not all of us will feel like the Grouch 48 hours before our period.

"If I didn't have that map of my experience across the course of the menstrual cycle, I would be... lost," Maisie Hill says. "I think many people are. Whereas, when we know it's a cycle, we can think: 'Of course I feel this way! I've got no hormone! I'm going to feel differently in a few days, no biggie.' As opposed to: 'I'm just so useless, I'm awful, why do

I feel this way? No one else feels this way!'"

Feeling hormonal, Maisie Hill goes on, is not just about our periods. It's about all the other hormonal cycles, including the daily release of melatonin, cortisol, thyroid-stimulating hormone, on which our circadian rhythm, our natural oscillations in mood and energy levels, and sleep–wake cycles entirely depend. "People wake up: it might take them a while to get going but, once they do, they hit that peak of feeling good and productive. But then, maybe there's the afternoon slump… they have an afternoon cup of tea and pick things up again, then towards the end of the day they want to wind down, finish things up and go to bed… We don't judge that AT ALL. No problem with it. But the menstrual cycle is something we associate with being female primarily – of course there are non-binary people, and trans people who have cycles – but because it's this 'Female Thing', it's viewed completely differently."

As unknowable? Unreliable? Sketchy? Silly?

"Untrustworthy. Unreliable. Reactive. Out of control."

That's so irritating!

"Highly."

WHEN THE MENSTRUAL CYCLE GOES WRONG

When it's working exactly as it should be, doing everything it should do, at the point it's supposed to do it, the menstrual cycle is a raucous, demanding sort of a proposition. Forceful and compelling and capable of causing all manner of trouble, of affecting our lives and our experiences and our emotional responses.

But when it goes wrong, which it does, for lots and lots of us? When it misfires or messes up or stops firing altogether? When it turns against us for reasons we cannot fathom? The pain and the trauma and the long-term impacts on our health can be extraordinary.

Andrew Horne is professor of gynaecology and reproductive sciences at the University of Edinburgh, a medic and scientist specialising in the diagnosis and treatment of endometriosis. He's also one of those profoundly calm, patient people, the sort who somehow make you want to cry, because they're *that* gentle, *that* unjudgementally interested in you. Professor Horne gets extra points for doing all that over Zoom.

"I think people think of the menstrual cycle as the period itself, quite naturally, because as a woman, that has a huge impact on your life, rather than, the process that's maybe in the lead up to the period," he tells me.

I certainly did, I say; but then I started talking to you lot.

"When you were a teenager, and you had your first period: do you think you were prepared for it? Or was it a terrifying experience? Sorry. I shouldn't be asking you questions."

It wasn't terrifying for me, no. I don't remember technically being prepared – presumably, my mum said something, school said something, I can't remember anything specific – but I knew exactly what was happening to me somehow, and that it was OK, normal. I guess I'd read *Are You There, God? It's Me, Margaret*, the Judy Blume book in which the lead character gets her first period; I certainly wasn't the first or the last of my school mates, so according to the research, it wouldn't have been a traumatic experience for me, on those grounds. I definitely didn't think I was dying, or anything like that.

What about when they go "wrong"? What does that mean, to you?

"When menstruation is heavy, painful. Understanding what's

normal. Knowing when to seek help."

Right, so: what is "normal"?

"A normal period is one that doesn't interfere with your ability to function – to work or study, or to engage socially. An abnormal period is one that stops you from doing those things. If you have to spend a day in bed, or if you're embarrassed to go out because you're bleeding heavily, or you're needing to take excessive amounts of painkillers. It's quite a subjective way of looking at it. In the past, people used to talk about volumes of blood and a cut-off being normal and abnormal. But that was shown, quite clearly, in research back in the 80s, that it didn't correspond with the impact it had on people's quality of life."

Because the amount of blood you lose does not necessarily correlate with the amount of pain you feel?

"No. So you can have a painless, very heavy bleed, and vice versa: you can have pain with minimal bleeding. And you can have pain at other times of your menstrual cycle: pain with ovulation, pain in the lead-up to menstruation, which can be incredibly impactful. They don't always sit together. People do have very painful, heavy periods, that is something that happens. But they can happen in isolation as well."

And what is endometriosis? I've heard the word, most generally in association with the celebrities who suffer from it, and who've talked about that: Chrissy Teigen, Alexa Chung, Emma Bunton, Lena Dunham... I know it's painful, and uterus related. But that's where I peak.

I learn that endometriosis is defined by the presence of tissue exactly like that found in the lining of the womb in other parts of the body. The most common place for endometrial tissue is within the pelvis, but, Professor Horne tells me, you can find endometriosis in places as remote as the lung. People who present with endometriosis in the lung often have pain which coincides with their menstrual cycle; they may well have a cyclical pattern of pain located in their chest, one which coincides with period pain, or "they might cough up blood".

"Superficial peritoneal" endometriosis, which occurs on the lining of the wall of the pelvis, accounts for about 80% of what Professor Horne sees. "Or you can have it on the ovaries, which causes cysts. People talk about 'chocolate cysts': they're called 'chocolate' because they've got altered blood inside them, which is brown in colour. Or they can have nodules of endometriosis, which often involve the bowel and the bladder and scar tissue." It hurts, because that tissue reacts to your hormonal shifts as if it were in the uterus; it thickens, bleeds, sheds, thickens, bleeds sheds: but it doesn't go anywhere. Your body might fight back against it, try to eliminate it with an inflammatory response designed to destroy it, which it doesn't; it only increases the pain. Endometriosis tissue can grow directly onto nerves, causing yet more extraordinary pain. It can lead to the formation of scar tissue (more pain). If it's in the bowel, it can cause obstructions, which can result in medical emergency, a threat to life – and that's just some of it. I click on the #endowarrior hashtag on Instagram and find countless women detailing their extraordinary endometriosis-related pain ("My ribs are hurting, even my face is swollen, I have pain shooting down my legs and into my back... I don't want to live here anymore, in this hell,") and sharing pictures of their #endobellies, exposed stomachs swollen, distended to three times the normal size by the condition.

All of this would be dismal in a rare condition, right? Unthinkable, really. Intolerable, unacceptable.

But endometriosis is not at all rare.

"Oh no. It's incredibly common," Professor Horne says.

"One in 10 people who menstruate can potentially have endometriosis. That's 200 million people worldwide."

Are all those people in terrible pain?

"No. Half the people who have endometriosis lesions may not experience symptoms at all, or at least, not significant symptoms. But there's a really wide range [of pain levels experienced]. The people I see, it's really impactful. It's affecting their relationships, their work. They really find it difficult to function."

Bloody hell.

"Yeah. So there are three big challenges with it. Understanding why it happens..."

How the tissue gets there in the first place?

"That's the million-dollar question. There are lots of theories. The oldest theory is that it's due to retrograde menstruation: when the menstrual tissue goes back up the fallopian tubes and into the pelvis. You see that in around 80–90 % of people who menstruate: some of it goes back. So the big question is: is that a contributing factor, and if it is, why does it stick and form the endometriosis lesions in some people and not others? We've done some work looking at the role of lactate – that's a chemical that's produced as a by-product of breaking down sugars. There is more lactate in the pelvis of people with endometriosis, compared with the pelvis of patients without. So we wonder whether lactate stimulates that process of developing the lesions. But there are other factors that are important as well. We know endometriosis is inherited. Twin studies have shown it runs in families, but what we haven't been able to do is identify a gene, or combination of genes, which predicts you're going to develop endometriosis."

There are Professor Horne tells me, various other theories about why endometriosis develops, none of which are conclusive.

The second big challenge is: how do you diagnose it?

"At the moment, it has to be diagnosed largely by keyhole surgery, by an operation, because it's not often seen on scans, and there isn't a blood test that can pick it up." Within months of my conversation with Professor Horne, in July 2023, news of a possible urine test for endometriosis broke. That test is in the process of being validated. As things stand, with laparoscopy, keyhole surgery, providing the only real method to diagnose endometriosis, sufferers in the UK wait an average of eight years to find out if they have it. "If you go to your GP and say, 'I'm getting really painful periods, it's impacting my quality of life,' they can't immediately say you have endometriosis… Sometimes, on a scan, you can pick up the cystic forms, but quite often patients end up being referred to hospital for keyhole surgery. The benefit of keyhole surgery to diagnose it is that the tissue can be removed at that time if it's straightforward. But in some cases, it's not."

Professor Horne says that some cases of endometriosis are "picked up" during infertility investigations. "We know that about a third of people with endometriosis will have difficulty conceiving. Sometimes it's picked up when a woman undergoes sterilisation… People don't tend to get laparoscopic sterilisation [where the fallopian tubes are clipped to prevent fertilisation of the eggs] very commonly now, but perhaps they've had a sterilisation procedure and the doctor's said: 'Actually, did you know you have endometriosis?' And some people don't realise they have it at all. We tend not to treat it in these cases. We only tend to treat it if it's causing symptoms."

Which brings him to the third major challenge concerning endometriosis: "We don't have a cure for it."

Sh*t.

"Broadly speaking, it's treated by surgery to remove or destroy the disease. But that doesn't work for everybody, and in some people who it does work for, the symptoms come back. On average, about 50% of people who benefit from surgery will have a recurrence of symptoms after around five years. So that's a challenge. And the treatments all rely on giving hormones to suppress the production of oestrogen from your ovaries, because we know oestrogen stimulates endometriosis."

Why?

"We don't know. Oestrogen is one of the sex hormones that causes endometrial cells to proliferate, to grow, so there are a number of factors that are important for endometriosis to survive and develop. The trouble with having to give hormones to people is, first of all, these treatments only work when you're taking them; secondly, hormones often have side effects. And also, this is a young population who maybe don't want to take hormones because they want to get pregnant."

I've learned enough by the time I speak to Professor Horne to appreciate that suppressing oestrogen is not useful when you're in the baby-making business, when you're trying to get pregnant – because it's a contraceptive.

Endometriosis can also be managed with medication alone – contraceptive pills or patches, or the Mirena coil, which also works by deploying hormones. In extreme cases, where medication or surgery, to physically cut the endometriosis tissue out of the parts of your body in which it's accumulated, don't work, the only option is a hysterectomy, i.e. complete removal of the uterus. However, this is a drastic recourse – a major surgery that puts the patient in menopause, assuming they weren't already in it, leaves her infertile and doesn't even guarantee the end of the pain. This makes the fact that I see some of the women using the #endowarrior hashtag on Instagram also posting about how seriously they're contemplating having hysterectomies more distressing yet.

There are movements in the understanding of endometriosis, however, not least due to the passion and graft of people like Professor Horne.

"I've worked on it for about 12 to 13 years now. I always remember going to see a mentor and saying I wanted to start working on it, and they said: 'This is really difficult, there's been no progress for years…' Almost trying to put me off. There still needs to be a lot more progress. But I have seen a change."

He says endometriosis gets nowhere near the funding it deserves, mainly due to the fact that funding panels have been historically comprised of men, which means that a much greater proportion of funding goes into diseases like diabetes, which affect both sexes, than endometriosis, which affects only women. However, he has started to see some progress recently.

"Awareness of endometriosis has increased, people like you are talking about it and that helps in raising awareness for research funding, raising awareness even within the hospital setting, that this is a problem, an issue, raising awareness among politicians, et cetera." This means understanding of the condition is evolving. Doctors used to think that endometriosis was a disease of women in their 30s and 40s, he tells me, but it can develop from the onset of menstruation. Because of the whole normalisation of pain in teenagers, people didn't think it was necessary to investigate further.

Because, being a woman = pain, so suck it up?

"Yeah. Which I hope is changing. You still hear stories of that. But also, this reluctance of doctors, because it means surgery, to make the diagnosis. To investigate. People saying: 'Oh we shouldn't be doing laparoscopies on teenagers. Actually, you are then denying them treatment, support, et cetera, et cetera." Early recognition of endometriosis is, he says, incredibly important because "while we don't know if it's a progressive disease, we *do* know that if you recognise endometriosis and treat the pain, it stops what we call the chronification of the pain. It stops it going from an acute pain to chronic pain."

I look up the difference between acute pain and chronic pain in the National Library of Medicine, the American database on medicine. It reads: "Acute pain is provoked by a specific disease or injury, serves a useful biological purpose, is associated with skeletal muscle spasm and sympathetic nervous system activation, and is self-limited. Chronic pain, in contrast, may be considered a disease state. It is pain that outlasts the normal time of healing, if associated with a disease or injury."

Professor Horne explains that chronic pain is much more difficult to manage. This is because the longer anyone suffers from pain, the more likely they are to become hypersensitive, to develop pain elsewhere in their body. The closest I've come to experiencing anything like this was when I injured that disc in my lower spine during Covid. I remember the pain going on for so long, it started to feel as if it owned me; I couldn't remember a time I didn't feel pain; it was almost as if I *was* my pain. And I probably experienced this for around six weeks to two months, max. With endometriosis, women experience pain for years and years and years; which means their bodies become more sensitive to pain – all and any pain – the longer that original pain continues. They can begin to experience intense pain anywhere in their bodies – not just in their pelvis, where it began.

"People with endometriosis often develop other types of pain," Professor Horne says. "Fibromyalgia, which is when you get pain all over your body. Or chronic migraines."

I wonder if this is emotional or physical; he tells me that it's both. Patients will get a whole range of pain symptoms, in addition to which they may suffer from lethargy and chronic tiredness. Next come the mental health problems, somewhat inevitable when you're living with chronic pain. You can feel isolated, become depressed. Yet another problem is that the neural pathways associated with pain, and those associated with mood management, sit very closely together in the brain. Consequently, not only does the experience of pain, unsurprisingly, affect your mood, but also your mood affects how you tolerate pain.

"Inflammation starts the pain process," Professor Horne tells me. This means that the swelling and build-up of tissue put pressure on nerve endings, which send pain signals to the brain. "But over a period of time, the nervous system becomes damaged. It makes your body perceive pain in a different way to how it should."

So it follows that the earlier endometriosis is recognised, diagnosed and treated, the better the chance a patient's pain will not progress from acute to chronic. Whether it does or not,

Professor Horne thinks clinical psychologists play an important part in how endometriosis patients are treated. "Previously, I think people felt if you were seeing a clinical psychologist, it was because the doctor thought [the pain] was all in your head. But actually, just acknowledging the major impact pain can have on your mood helps; also, acknowledging there are certain things you can do to improve your pain."

For example?

"Mindfulness. Pacing."

Pacing?

"A lot of patients with endometriosis, or any chronic pain conditions, have this boom-or-bust way of behaving. As soon as they feel they're not in pain, they go out and do lots and lots of things, then come back – and they're in agony for days. So it's kind of making people aware of that, and trying to stop them, when they are going through a good phase, from overdoing it."

Professor Horne goes on to talk about adenomyosis, another condition specifically affecting women, which had recently been in the press because the BBC newsreader Naga Munchetty had talked about her experience of it. He tells me that adenomyosis is similar to endometriosis in terms of the symptoms, but the cause is different: it's what happens when tissue from the womb's lining grows into its muscular wall. It can only be diagnosed with very careful imaging.

"For a long time, it was only diagnosed once a woman had undergone a hysterectomy. When that womb was looked at in the lab, they would see that the patient had adenomyosis. It's probably as common as endometriosis. We just don't know very much about it. It's very difficult to manage because the tissue is stuck within the muscle in the wall of the womb, so we can't easily cut it out, to remove it. Patients tend to have either surgery to remove the whole of the womb – but that's not suitable for everybody – or they have to rely on the hormone treatment."

It sounds like there are a lot of women out there in a lot of pain.

"A lot of the figures we have are based on estimates. We're trying to do some work with Denmark, where we're looking at questionnaire data to try and find out a bit more about how common these symptoms are, to have a bit more objective information. I think people hide pain a lot. Some people are very accepting that that's just them."

I wonder about the idea, narrative, even, that women experience more pain than men, and that this is somehow our lot, that we're "built for it", as a man once said to me at a party, as if a propensity for enduring pain is the female equivalent of a car specification on us.

What's the truth in that from Professor Horne's perspective?

"I think absolutely. The menstrual cycle, pregnancy are painful experiences. I think there's no doubt. Do you not?"

I don't know. If I think about it, it makes sense.

"Migraine is more common in women." Three times more likely, according to pretty much all available research, plus we experience them more frequently. I'm one of those female migraine sufferers, I should know.

As for this idea that women somehow manage pain better, are built for it: "I think women are very accepting of pain. Particularly in relation to menstruation, but also in relation to things like migraines."

"I feel like women almost get on with it, try and deal with it. And that's good in some ways, but often, they're missing out on help and treatments that might make their lives much more bearable. I think it must be awful living in pain the whole time. Or managing pain, managing your life around the pain, which I think a lot of people do. I do feel, with the women I see often: how have you coped with this? How have you put up with it for so long?"

And it isn't just about pain, he tells me. There's also the terrible impact on relationships, as well as on the ability to socialise. Sex can be very painful, plus about a third of endometriosis patients are affected by infertility. In spite of this, Professor Horne says, "I'm always quite positive with patients when they get their initial diagnosis. In two-thirds of cases, people have no difficulty getting pregnant, and actually, even in the third, if you do have to go for something like IVF, often endometriosis patients respond well."

Which is cheering.

ANOTHER WAY PERIODS GO WRONG

"A way to think about periods," says Professor Hilary Critchley, a ferociously direct, fathomlessly smart individual, who tells me she's glad I'm recording her, less chance I'll get things wrong (though not zero chance – she's met journalists before), "is as the most brilliant, normal physiological example of a wound that heals without scarring every month." Bleed, then heal, bleed, then heal? "Yes. It's quite incredible, the way the body is orchestrated, so it can do that perfectly. But when you upset something, that's what we need to understand more about."

Professor Critchley is a clinician and an academic: a clinical academic. For the last 30 years, her work has been focussed on gynaecology, particularly periods. "The topic of bleeding problems. Rather than period *pain*." Pain, she tells me, can accompany heavy bleeding, although not always.

She first became interested in periods 40 years ago. Back then, she says: "It was a taboo area." And now? "I think that's where the tragedy is." She tells me that 20 years after her academic study began, she gave her inaugural lecture on the topic, during which she talked about how it is not sufficiently addressed. "Twenty years after that? *Now*? The patients I see, research I do – I sum it up as: under-recognised, under-researched and under-resourced."

Still taboo, effectively?

"Yes. People don't like talking about bleeding. Society doesn't like talking about it. But if I were to say to you, one in three has bleeding problems, and even that is probably an underestimate…"

Well, then: bleeding is something that needs to be talked about, and desperately.

What does it mean to have "bleeding problems"? What qualifies as a problem?

"I do this bench science… We use this phrase: 'bench to bedside and back again.'"

The bench is the laboratory, the bedside is the patient; the phrase describes the clinical academic's experience, the division of their time between patients and their real-life issues, and the development of treatments, which can help with those issues.

"You collect period products, and you extract the blood, measure the amount of blood – that's what we do. If I told you some of our patients lose the equivalent of: imagine you were a blood donor, every month…"

That's... a pint? We give a pint of blood when we donate, no?
"Yes."

Some women are losing *that much*?

"Yes. Normal is about a small egg cup – so imagine losing a pint of blood a month! I have the most wonderful team of research nurses, and they go out to the homes, or the patients bring in their collections, and these would be really heavy bags [of blood-sodden period products]. And the graphic descriptions people bring into the clinic. They bring their phones in and show me pictures [of their blood loss], because they think: 'Oh, the doctor will never believe me'. I can well believe it. We've measured it, we've seen it."

How does this impact the lives of women?

"We're sitting here – imagine you're terrified that when you get up... the fear of getting up from a seat and leaving it stained."

TBH, I've had moments like that over the years – multiple. Hadn't occurred to me before that it wasn't, you know, just kinda how things go...

"You're never going to wear white." Yup, been there too, opted for the black jeans, for safety's sake... "You will not leave the house."

Ah, no, it never got me that bad.

"I have stories where their job is threatened. 'I've got to have something done about this, because I'm having too many days off work. I'm going to lose my job...' One of the commonest causes of anaemia, that is not recognised, is heavy periods. Iron deficiency."

I'd read that almost 35% of American women under 50 are

iron deficient,[24] I tell Professor Critchley. Is that true?

"I think it's far more prevalent than we are aware. The World Health Organization wants to reduce it worldwide by 50%. They're looking at diet, infection, other things that may be causing it – but there's very little mention of heavy menstruation as a cause. It's my next big thing to address. Because, if you're iron deficient when you go into pregnancy, you're at higher risk of poorer pregnancy outcomes. It can also affect your infant. It can be transgenerational… [If] you've had heavy periods for 30 years, you're iron deficient and you go into menopause, is your brain fog there because you're menopausal, or because you're grossly iron deficient?"

So if our iron levels are low, do you think supplements are the way to go?

"Yes, we should consider it if our periods are heavy and impacting daily life, such as feeling tired all the time too. Bottom line is, we normalise heavy periods too much and so may not be aware that a period is heavy, and we don't recognise the other wider impacts on health. We need to not normalise it [in periods]."

There are nine causes of "abnormal uterine bleeding", heavy periods. Hilary Critchley was one of three clinical scientists who, in 2011, developed a classification for it, alongside Professors Malcolm Munro, based in the US, and Ian Fraser, based in Australia.

---

24 More than a third of women under 50 are iron-deficient, *New York Times*, 2023 – https://www.nytimes.com/2023/10/17/well/live/iron-deficiency-symptoms-women.html

"It's called the PALM-COEIN[25] classification of abnormal uterine bleeding. It's now used all over the world. Look at your palm. Think of a coin, on your palm."

I do.

Professor Critchley then goes on to explain what the acronym means. The PALM bit is all the structural causes that might give you abnormal bleeding, things that can be seen with a scan. **P is for polyp,** a local thickness in the womb lining; **A is for adenomyosis,** which, as we've learned, is endometrial tissue growing within the muscle in the wall of the womb; **L is for leiomyoma,** which is another word for fibroids – non-cancerous growths that develop in the wall of the womb, which can be the size of a pea, or a melon, and anywhere in between; and **M is for malignancy** – this can be an early sign of problems in the womb lining.

The COEIN bit, meanwhile, is the causes you *can't* see. To diagnose these, Professor Critchley, says, "You have to have time to talk to your patients, delve deeper."

Abnormal bleeding in a COEIN situation might be a consequence of: **C, which stands for coagulopathy,** "bleeding disorders", conditions which prevent your blood clotting effectively, and which are generally inherited. "There's one called Von Willebrand. If you have Von Willebrand, your periods are going to be heavy from the moment they start." **O is for ovulatory disorders,** when you don't ovulate regularly, meaning you get too long an exposure to oestrogen. You have very irregular periods, but when they come, they are very heavy.

---

25 The two FIGO systems for normal and abnormal uterine bleeding symptoms and classification of causes of abnormal uterine bleeding in the reproductive years, *Int J Gynaecol Obstet*, 2018 – https://doi.org/10.1002/ijgo.12666

Why would you not ovulate?

"Polycystic ovaries. Sometimes stress. Extreme athletic activity. Body weight. Sometimes, you're just born someone who doesn't ovulate regularly." Both excessively high or low BMI can increase the risk of anovulation. According to my experts, it's increasingly common for people to overexercise or undereat to the point of losing their periods.

E is for endometrial, problems relating to the lining of the womb. "We don't understand it enough. That's the research I do at the bench, " says Professor Critchley. **I is Iatrogenic** – this refers to any illness resulting from medical examination or treatment. "There's lots of things we do that can disturb our bleeding pattern. Any form of hormone: if you've got a [contraceptive] implant, if you're on a depo injection [the contraceptive injection], if you've got a hormone-releasing coil in the womb cavity, if you're taking a combined contraceptive, if you're taking the progesterone-only pill… Whatever route, whatever preparation, whatever regime: 20% of hormone therapy users will experience unscheduled bleeding. We don't understand it. It's a class effect of hormones." Another Iatrogenic cause might be taking an anticoagulant drug like warfarin, which is often prescribed, if you've had a blood clot in your chest or leg, for example. This would make you have heavy periods.

"Even some antidepressants will interfere with your ovulation," says Professor Critchley.

Because they affect the hypothalamus which also controls ovulation?

"Exactly! They affect the control pathways. It's not that they are causing heavier bleeds; they're indirectly causing it because they're interfering with normal ovulation." Having said which, antidepressants shouldn't be abandoned suddenly, and never without discussion with a doctor.

Finally, the **N is for not otherwise classified,** which can include incredibly rare conditions like uterine arteriovenous malformation, "an abnormal connection between uterine arteries and vein." The point *is*, Professor Critchley says, accurate diagnosis involves an incredibly delicate, detailed and nuanced conversation with your patient, one which revolves around the individual, their history, their medication, their needs, their desires. Their fears.

How to establish which of the nine causes we're dealing with? I learn from Professor Critchley that the visible causes, the PALM, are diagnosed by ultrasound, a scan, which uses sound-waves to create an image of some interior part of the body, or by pipelle. A pipelle is a fine plastic straw around two millimetres in diameter, with a removable central section. When that centre is removed, it creates a negative pressure; this means that when introduced into the cavity of the womb, the pipelle will suck out a sample of the womb lining. This sample can then be sectioned and looked at under a microscope to check whether it is normal or not. Professor Critchley says she would do this for anybody in a high-risk group to exclude changes in the lining of the womb, which might later develop into endometrial (womb lining) cancer. She explains that high-risk groups in the UK, as reflected in clinical guidelines, may include women aged 45 years and over, while in other countries the lower age limit is 40. She also says she believes it's not entirely useful to work to rigid cut-offs like this. If her patient had a higher BMI (body mass index), and she was only 39, she advises taking a sample with a pipelle, because a higher BMI can be associated with increased endometrial cancer risks.

If neither ultrasound scans, nor pipelle samples, nor MRI imaging provide sufficient information on what is causing a patient's abnormal bleeding, then, Professor Critchley tells me, you can assume you're dealing with causes from the COEIN group of issues – the things that cannot be seen. At this point, conversations begin, on your medical history, that of your family, on the medications you take or have taken historically, and for what.

Treatment varies according to diagnosis, and different approaches work better, depending on the root cause of your bleeding, which is why you've got to get it right.

Professor Critchley says it's a bit like going through a menu of treatments. You work your way through, and maybe, in the end, the patient says she's had enough and just wants it all taken away.

I'd read somewhere that heavy bleeding is the main reason a third of women aged between 30 and 49 get hysterectomies, I say.

She replies that it is at least that figure. The aim is to get the diagnosis right first time, to reduce that dissatisfaction and the number of hysterectomies. "To me, when you're presenting the patient with the menu, hysterectomy is at the bottom. I believe it should be at the bottom. It's a massive decision for anybody, there are risks, and if we can find an alternative, we should be trying to." It's worth mentioning that hysterectomy rates for heavy bleeding have dropped in recent years, thanks to better treatment options. Often, doctors will suggest trying the combined contraceptive pill or a hormone-releasing coil (like the progesterone IUS), as these options can make a big difference and are far less invasive.

So what's above hysterectomy on the menu?

"In the UK, we tend to start with medical options. The hypothalamus, the pituitary, they talk to each other, produce messages which go into the blood and talk to the ovaries. The ovaries produce the oestrogen and the progesterone; those two hormones work in the womb, on the lining of the womb… And the fibroids, if they're there."

Aha! So oestrogen and progesterone make fibroids grow?

"Oestrogen does. When you get to menopause, unless you take hormone replacement therapy (HRT), the fibroids may get smaller," because they're deprived of oestrogen. "You can reproduce that in a younger woman with a monthly injection. They've used that for 40 years."

What's in the injection?

"It's called gonadotropin-releasing hormone analogue. It switches off the hypothalamic-pituitary-ovarian conversation. You will have all the symptoms of menopause. That's the downside. The upside is, your fibroids will not grow, they may get smaller. Though for reasons we don't understand, not everyone responds. But most do."

But the patient is in menopause?

"Yes, but it's reversible." There is a concern that, over time, the symptoms of young women experiencing menopause-related hormone loss could be damaging, "So you have to work with the patient. After a certain number of months, you'd try and give a little bit of oestrogen back, help the oestrogen deficiency symptoms, the sweats, the flushes. You also don't want to have bone loss brought on too early.

"In the last 12 months, rather than an injection, there is now a daily oral tablet, designed to have the same effect. This tablet has a small dose of hormone replacement in it. It will stop the bleeding, but because you've got a small dose of hormone replacement, it's not quite as effective as the injection alone in reducing the fibroid size."

If a patient is hoping to get pregnant while experiencing "problematic periods", placing them in temporary, medical menopause is obviously not an option.

"Then, we're only left with two options, and they're the same ones we had when I started my training. One of them involves haemostasis, which is about helping blood to clot." Haemostasis is the process by which our bodies close off any wound, from a paper cut onwards. "There's a particular drug called tranexamic acid, which you only take for the four or five days when you're having your period. There are a lot of myths about it."

Tranexamic acid has been linked to blood clots, aka haemostasis in overdrive, when there is far too much clotting, dangerous amounts of it, and the body is left at risk of heart attack, stroke or pulmonary embolism. However, according to the NHS website, serious side effects relating to the use of tranexamic acid such as dangerous clots "are rare and happen in less than one in 1,000 people."[26] Professor Critchley says: "Millions of women have used it for four decades. The risks are extremely small, and it is an extremely effective non-hormonal treatment for reducing period blood loss." All other

---

26 Side effects of tranexamic acid, NHS, 2025 – https://www.nhs.uk/medicines/tranexamic-acid/side-effects-of-tranexamic-acid/

approaches involve some sort of hormone control, she adds: "Which is why we need new approaches."

Professor Critchley and I discuss the issue Professor Horne raised, about how pain, once it becomes chronic, sensitises us to other kinds of pain, which can mean that ultimately, our pain may not even be coming from the womb. This means that, while Professor Critchley's last-choice treatment option of hysterectomy will always end bleeding problems – no womb, no blood – it won't necessarily end pain.

"We can't make that promise."

I ask Professor Critchley what she wants now, 40 years into her noble, bold, taboo-busting endeavour; how we go forward with diagnosis and treatment of abnormal uterine bleeding. She says she wants more funding, more research, more treatments; "more personalised approaches. We need education around menstruation, so if periods are heavy, they don't become normalised. Late primary. Secondary. For everyone. Not just those who menstruate. Everybody.

"One thing that's really important," she continues, "we need to stop describing – whether it's menstrual pain, whether it's horrendous periods – we need to stop describing them as 'benign conditions'. We need to describe these conditions as 'chronic, debilitating'. Yes, these are not malignant. They are not cancerous. They're life altering, not life threatening – but they could become life threatening. If you're losing so much blood or you're at risk of a pulmonary embolism because you've got a big mass in your tummy."

But even if they're not – they're hardly "benign"?

"No. Not at all."

WHAT I KNOW NOW

- The menstrual cycle is about much more than "just periods". It involves daily hormonal shifts throughout the month, which can be broken down into four phases:
  Phase 1 – menstruation, when we experience blood loss, and when hormone levels are very low.
  Phase 2 – the follicular phase, during which our levels of oestradiol begin to rise.
  Phase 3 – ovulation, during which our levels of oestradiol, LH and FSH are at their highest.
  Phase 4 – the luteal phase, when progesterone becomes dominant.

- Every last one of these phases can impact our mood, negatively or positively. For example, as oestrogen peaks, ovulation can leave you feeling super confident and gregarious, and more likely to indulge in risky behaviour.

- Each phase can also affect performance. Phase 4, the luteal phase, is often the most precarious in terms of injury – although this can vary from woman to woman.

- Hormones also affect our ability to process alcohol and nicotine. E.g. Women are more likely to feel the impact of alcohol – to feel drunker, quicker – when we're ovulating.

- One in 10 women has endometriosis, a painful condition in which womb lining tissue is shed into other parts of the body (usually within the pelvis), causing inflammation.

- As many as one in three women experiences menstrual bleeding so heavily that it creates problems for them.

- The usual amount of blood lost during a period is roughly a small eggcupful, which is admittedly hard to assess... But, you know! As a guide.

CHAPTER FOUR

WHAT'S A VAGINA?

Before I learned that the vagina came under the "primary sex characteristic umbrella" – which was two chapters ago – I definitely thought I knew what a vagina was.

Everyone knows, eh?

It's the thing.

The very centre of femaleness. The heart of it. The heat of it.

And it is naughty and rude and sacred and divine, depending on context and whom you ask.

I knew that!

I also knew about vajazzles – the practice, fashionable in the 2010s, of decorating the female pubic area with stick-on jewels. I knew about Brazilians – the removal of all or most pubic hair, because that is what social trends, most likely inspired by the aesthetic of pornography, demand. I knew from experience that a dose of thrush, a common yeast infection, can usually be sorted out with a smearing of natural yoghurt. I knew about vibrators, and that Gwyneth Paltrow advocates the inserting of jade "Yoni" eggs into vaginas for healing purposes (she sells them on her website Goop for US$66).[27]

---

27 Jade Egg, Goop Wellness, https://goop.com/
goop-wellness-jade-egg/p/?srsltid=AfmBOooTY1BV8OFTjuvwkuYtbHVaja
7o-C76AN5CoZVh0-s2twkBlnH6

I knew the essentials, right?

Guess what?

I didn't.

I knew virtually nothing. Nor do you.

Time to speak to some experts.

What exactly is a vagina? I ask Dr Alison Wright, consultant obstetrician and gynaecologist at the Portland Hospital, where she serves as vice chair of the medical advisory committee; she also works as an obstetrician and gynaecologist in the NHS, based at the Royal Free Hospital in north London.

"That," she replies, "is a surprisingly difficult question." She's a quietly, carefully spoken women who is also – forgive me, it's my fash-mag training – *incredibly* well dressed. I've already enquired as to the origins of her shoes, already established that This Gynaecologist Wears Prada.

Back to vaginas.

"First of all," Dr Wright says, "I feel very strongly that we should talk about 'vaginas'. The word. Women coming to see me as patients will sometimes talk about 'down below'. And I know they talked like that with their GP [too]. 'Down below'. 'Down there'. A lot of people don't know what a bladder is…"

(The urinary bladder is a temporary storage reservoir for urine, located in the pelvic cavity. It is not your vagina.)

"And they don't know what the pelvic floor is…"

(The pelvic floor muscles support the bladder, uterus and bowel; they are not your vagina either – though they are incredibly important to it; we'll return to them.)

So: if we're not calling things by their actual names, if we're not distinguishing between organs and even muscle groups, how can we know what's hurting us? What isn't working? How can we communicate it to doctors, if we think of it just as one amorphous mass, labelled, vaguely, "down there"?

"Yes! Just call it the 'vagina'. If you're 'bleeding from somewhere down there' it might be rectal bleeding."

It might be your foot, to be fair.

"It might. So: the vagina."

Yes!

"It's the passage between the womb and the outside."

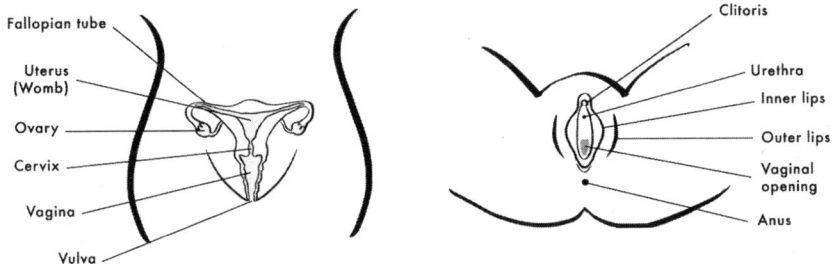

"Oh, we *really* need to teach women and girls this," says Dr Shazia Malik, a consultant obstetrician and gynaecologist who's worked in women's health for over 30 years. I arrange to interview her to talk about her sub-specialism: reproductive health and infertility, but when I raise the topic of vaginas – in a very nice cake shop near her consulting rooms – ouf! Her face lights up like fireworks.

"Can we talk about them? They're one of my pet subjects!"

There's a substantial lack of vagina-knowledge out there, huh, I say.

"Yes! But you can't blame women for that! We need to give

women the information, really, that they should have got at school."

Like?

"'This is what your vagina can do! This is where it *is*! This is what keeps your vagina healthy. What is your vulva? How is that different to your vagina?'"

The vulva, as per the diagram on the previous page, is the outside bit of your genitalia, the visible bits, the labia, the tip of your clitoris – but *only* the tip, I'll learn from Dr Philippa Kaye, whom I arrange to interview because she's particularly knowledgeable about breasts (Chapter 5), though it turns out she knows a thing or two about vaginas, too.

"When people think of the clitoris, they think of a little nobble," Dr Kaye will tell me literally moments after we say hello. "Actually, that little nobble is like the tip of a nose. It's got what looks like legs and bulbs, which extend down in the vulva, and fill with blood during arousal, like a penis fills with blood during arousal. That's why most women will not reach orgasm from penetration alone. Because they need that whole area stimulated."

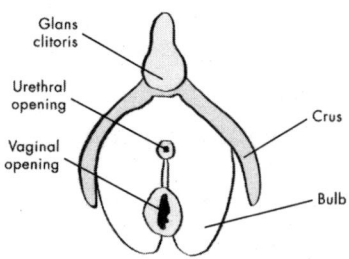

Glans clitoris

Urethral opening

Vaginal opening

Crus

Bulb

"Where is your cervix?" asks Dr Malik.

Top of the vagina, entrance to the womb? I ask.

I'm right!

"Why should you have the HPV vaccine?" she goes on.

That I don't know. It transpires that the HPV vaccine is the vaccine offered to all children – girls and, since 2019, boys – aged between 12 and 13 as part of the NHS vaccination programme. It protects against infection by certain types of human papillomavirus, the virus responsible for genital warts, and most forms of cervical cancer. Should you not get it at school, the vaccine is available on the NHS to women aged up to 25 years. "Did you know that?" Dr Malik asks me. I did not, I admit. After 25, both men and women can pay for it privately, up to the age of 45.

Why might you not have the HPV vaccine at school?

"If your mum says she's an anti-vaxxer [for example]. Does that mean you'll never have the HPV vaccine? Or would you like to read the information, and then, when you're an adult, you can make the decision for yourself?" Dr Malik says. "That may still be not to have the HPV vaccine…"

But at least you've got the info?

"Right."

What's the vagina made of? I ask Dr Alison Wright. "Mucosa: tissue," she says. Mucosa is a moist inner lining, which coats some organs and body cavities, the digestive and respiratory systems, for example, as well as the reproductive. This lining is attached to the vaginal muscles by fascia, connective tissue.

And what does it *do*?

"What is the *job* of the vagina?" asks Dr Malik. "Is it just there for you to have sex? Or to have babies? No!"

"It is to connect the outer world to your cervix, your womb, your fallopian tubes and your ovaries. It's an organ, a separate organ." Dr Malik explains that it changes during puberty, when it becomes proportionally larger. The vulva – that outer visible area – becomes covered in pubic hair, darker and more pigmented; then continues to change through the course of the reproductive life. During childbearing years, your vaginal mucosa responds to your hormonal cycle. It is at its thickest mid-cycle, around ovulation. In menopause, depleting oestrogen levels mean that it becomes less hydrated and more irritated, and the mucosa gets thinner. Until recently, that menopausal phase had been called "vaginal atrophy" – a term that's not only quite gross but also misleading, because it also affects tissues outside the vagina. It's now called GSM, genitourinary syndrome of menopause.

"So your vagina literally connects the outside world to the inside of your abdomen," Dr Malik goes on. "To your pelvis. Otherwise, how would a sperm meet an egg? When you have sex and there's a sperm… it has to get [up the vagina], through the cervix, swim up through your uterus – your womb – go through your fallopian tubes. Your fallopian tubes have to pick up an egg so that the sperm can meet the egg in the fallopian tube, right? This means that whatever is going on in your vagina can directly impact what is going on in your pelvis. Your vagina communicates with your pelvis."

And what does it… *say?*

She explains that it's not a question of *conversation*, so much as impact. If something goes wrong with the vagina, it follows that it might subsequently go wrong with the whole of the pelvis. For example:

"We tell girls sexually transmitted infections (STIs) are 'bad' – but why are they bad?"

I don't know!

As well as causing pain, bleeding after sex or between periods, and in extreme cases, pelvic inflammatory disease, "they can [also] make you infertile. If a sexual partner gives you a dose of chlamydia [a common bacterial STI spread by contact with infected genital fluids, vaginal fluids or semen], that can go through your cervix, into your uterus, through into your fallopian tubes. Your fallopian tubes have tiny little hairs inside them, which waft the egg and the sperm together. If you damage those little hairs – cilia, they're called – the fallopian tube can't do its job."

And as Dr Malik explains, cilia damage can sometimes have serious consequences: "So your dose of chlamydia has damaged those little cilia, which stops the egg meeting the sperm. But also, because they're damaged, if you did manage to get pregnant, if the sperm *did* meet the egg, the other job [of the cilia] is to transport that fertilised egg into your uterus. If it can't do that effectively, the egg implants in your fallopian tube, and you get an ectopic pregnancy."

An ectopic pregnancy is when a fertilised egg implants itself outside of the womb, usually in one of the fallopian tubes. This egg can't develop into a baby, and can put your health at serious risk, should the pregnancy continue.

As well as ectopic pregnancies, STIs can also cause PID – pelvic inflammatory disease – which can result in severe sepsis, pelvic adhesions and infertility as well as chronic pain.

An infection can also make the fallopian tubes dilate and fill with fluid, causing a blockage called a hydrosalpinx, which can make it harder to conceive.

"Did you know different STIs are increasing?" Dr Malik asks.

I did not!

"Yes. Chlamydia, gonorrhoea…"

Gonorrhoea?

"Yes!"

That's so… Victorian. Except apparently not; apparently it's very *now*. I find a UK government website which confirms: "gonorrhoea diagnoses increased to 82,592 in 2022, an increase of 50.3% compared to 2021 (54,961) and 16.1% compared to 2019 (prior to the Covid-19 pandemic) – this is the highest number of diagnoses in any one year since records began in 1918."[28] Also: "infectious syphilis diagnoses increased to 8,692 in 2022, up 15.2% compared to 2021 (7,543) and 8.1% compared to 2019 – this is the largest annual number since 1948."

"Did you know that you have peaks of STIs in girls in their late teens and early 20s?" Dr Malik asks me. "But then, when is the next biggest peak? In peri- and postmenopausal women! Because you know you don't need contraception. If you're on the apps, you're meeting somebody new, it is your absolute right and choice when you have sex. But if he's not had an STI screening, or even if he has, actually…"

It's important to use a condom, up until the point you can make a fully informed decision about not using one any more. Dr Malik is ferocious about empowering all women – the newly single 40- and 55-somethings, and teenage girls, and everyone in between, to demand male partners use a condom. The pressure on teenage girls is, she says, frightening – and all related to pornography and social media. She talks about the teenage girls

---

28 Gonorrhoea and syphilis at record levels in 2022, GOV.UK, 2023 – https://www.gov.uk/government/news/gonorrhoea-and-syphilis-at-record-levels-in-2022

who come to see her in her clinic, full of tales about how the boys in their school insist that oral sex is not really sex – when in fact HPV can be transmitted orally; as can syphilis and gonorrhoea.

"We're not teaching girls *that any kind of sexual contact is sex* [and we should be!]. As a gynaecologist, it's very easy to focus on women [and girls], but unless we educate the boys – unless we're going to schools and talking to boys *with* girls – about empowerment, what the consequences of unprotected sex are, why it can be harmful, all that stuff, then, *what are we doing?*"

She's ablaze.

I ask her what else she'd like people to know about the vagina, which is when she introduces me to a concept which I'd never heard of before, but which both instantly fascinates me and demands a section of its very own.

THE VAGINAL MICROBIOME

In the early 2020s, medical and wellness communities started to show huge interest in the gut microbiome, the microorganisms that populate our digestive tract and which are, it transpired, crucial to both men and women in terms of supporting many aspects of our health – our immune systems, mood and behaviours among them. There was much less discussion of the vaginal microbiome, an equivalent collection of microorganisms, located in the vagina. Ina Schuppe Koistinen, associate professor at the Karolinska Institutet in Sweden, and something of an expert in vaginal microbiome, describes it as "all the microbes that are present. That's bacteria, but also viruses, fungi and all kinds of single-cell organisms."

Like the gut microbiome, the vaginal microbiome has a significant impact on our overall health.

How healthy yours is depends on how well balanced it is, with specific reference to bacteria called *Lactobacilli*. *Lactobacilli* – particularly, a subset called *Lactobacillus crispatus* – is the main line of defence against infection. It can get disrupted by fragranced soaps and harsh detergents, which is why, Dr Malik says, we need to get rid of the idea that the vagina is somehow dirty. "We've got to kill that concept," she says.

The microbiome is responsible for the way vaginas smell. Dr Malik is passionate about telling young girls that their vaginas shouldn't *not* smell – they should have a healthy odour. This smell has been described as tangy, fermented, sour, or as metallic – like a jar of pennies – during menstruation, because of the iron present in blood.[29]

Dr Malik is vehemently anti-douche, the practice of washing your vagina with products. "You mustn't douche your vagina!" she says. "I'm forever saying: 'Use warm water to wash around your vulva. And just warm water…' But do wash with soap around your anus when you open your bowels, so you haven't got any of those gut bacteria lingering there on your panties waiting to get into your vagina."

Douches, Dr Malik adds, are not only a commercial con born of the misogynistically whiffy belief that vaginas are inherently dirty, and therefore any smell they produce is inherently unpleasant and unhealthy; they are also, potentially, actively dangerous.

---

29 Vaginal odor: what is normal?, *Moreland OB-GYN*, 2025 – https://www.morelandobgyn.com/blog/vaginal-odor-what-is-normal

She believes douches disrupt and destroy healthy vaginal micro-biome, and that they can even push an infection – an STI, should you be suffering from one – further up into the uterus, fallopian tubes and ovaries.

When your vaginal microbiome is out of balance, you can get infections like thrush. Thrush is a common yeast infection, which can affect both the vagina and the penis. It causes itchiness, irritation and a white, cottage cheese-y discharge. It's not an STI, it's generally harmless, but it can be uncomfortable; heaven knows, it once drove me half-crazy on a French exchange trip. At the same time, a healthy vagina will also have a discharge; it's how it cleans itself, among other things.

"Did you know your vaginal discharge changes through the menstrual cycle?" Dr Malik asks. I did not. "Mid-cycle, you get a thin watery discharge, because your body ovulates around mid-cycle. That's when you would get pregnant – if you were trying to get pregnant. That discharge changes to facilitate the sperm. To get it through the cervix."

No way! And yet, at the same time: *of course!*

Dr Malik says that many girls and women see this normal, healthy, *necessary* discharge and mistakenly think they have thrush. If the discharge has a strong, fishy smell, however, it could be BV, bacterial vaginosis, another indication your vaginal microbiome is disrupted. Like thrush, it isn't an STI. A lot of the time, discharges are, in fact, perfectly normal; it's just that we're not taught to recognise that, embrace the slight mess and whiff that just *is* a healthy vagina. Thrush treatment is available over the counter at high street chemists, but both expensive and pointless, if the woman buying it and using it doesn't actually have thrush. BV and thrush can only be accurately diagnosed by swab tests. It's important to get tested, particularly for BV, as it can be a risk factor for HPV (human papillomavirus) and CIN (Cervical intraepithelial neoplasia – the growth of abnormal cells on the cervix). [30,31]

As well as avoiding products and douches, there's evidence that steering clear of prolonged exposure to moist environments, such as hot tubs or baths, can protect against recurring UTIs, BV and thrush.[32]

According to a study published in 2024,[33] a healthy vaginal microbiome also plays a role in protecting against persistent UTIs, urinary tract infections. Studies have found that UTIs are 30 times more common in women than men, and that four in 10 women who suffer from them will get one at least once every six months.

Which is miserable.

This is believed to be because women have a shorter urethra (the channel between the bladder and the point where pee is released, your pee channel basically) than men, which means there's less distance for bacteria to travel, so more of them get up to your bladder and cause painful mayhem. That shorter urethra

---

30   A cross-sectional analysis about bacterial vaginosis, high-risk human papillomavirus infection, and cervical intraepithelial neoplasia in Chinese women, *Scientific Reports*, 2022 – https://www.nature.com/articles/s41598-022-10532-1
31   Association between bacterial vaginosis with human papillomavirus in the United States, *BMC Women's Health*, 2024 – https://doi.org/10.1186/s12905-024-02956-w
32   How to prevent a UTI: 19 do's and don'ts, King Edward VII's hospital, 2025 – https://www.kingedwardvii.co.uk/health-hub/how-to-prevent-uti-urinary-tract-infection
33   The role of the gut, urine, and vaginal microbiomes in the pathogenesis of urinary tract infection in women and consideration of microbiome therapeutics, *Open Forum Infectious Diseases*, 2024 – https://doi.org/10.1093/ofid/ofae471

also means that the anus, the bum and the entrance to the urethra are much closer to each other in women than men. For this reason, Dr Malik says we need to teach girls not to wear panties at night.

Really?

"Super important. The opening to your vagina is a few centimetres from your anus. Your gut is full of different bacteria to your vagina; so if you wear panties at night, any of the bacteria around your anus has a warm moist environment to proliferate."

Right there in your pants?

"In your panties! Then they can get into your vagina."

During the day, she says: "Wear cotton underwear as much as possible, don't teach [girls and women] that only slinky underwear, only G strings, are the thing!"

"Wash your underwear separate to your other clothes, at a high temperature. You can't kill the bacteria until you wash at 60–70 degrees. Thrush is a fungus – it will not die at low temperatures."

I had no clue and promptly overhaul my knicker-washing strategy.

Smoking, antibiotics, menstrual blood and exposure to other microbiome – those present in sperm, for example – can also disrupt a healthy microbiome, which is why we need to support it in every way we can.

THE PELVIC FLOOR

Remember I told you we'd get back to the pelvic floor muscles?

It's time.

And I know that, just reading those words alone, most of you have instantly, quietly started doing "Kegels" – tried to, anyway. Attempted what you imagine/hope/vaguely comprehend to be Kegels (named for Dr Arnold Kegel, the American gynaecologist who developed them, in the early- to mid-20th century); a kind of clenching, rhythmic gripping, contractions of something deep and inner, staccato tensing of the muscles you switch on when you're trying to stop yourself from farting or peeing. Kegels: which you know you're *supposed* to do, though you don't really know why? And you kind of think it's embarrassing? Because it's hidden and connected with your lower pelvis, which is always a little shame-laden? And because they're weird and not-quite-knowable and who can ever really say if you're doing them right because, what's the measure, and also: what's the point?

Dr Alison Wright tells me that the tissue that makes up the vagina lining, the mucosa, is surrounded by muscle and fascia. This, then, is the pelvic floor.

"It runs from our pubic bone to the coccyx," aka the tailbone, the nobbly bit at the very bottom of your spine, "which is where it attaches. It supports the vagina, and also the bladder neck, so it's quite low down. It also supports around the anus, the back passage. I demonstrate it like this…"

Dr Wright makes a cradle of her hands.

"It cradles the bladder neck at the front, the vagina in the middle, and your anus, at the end."

A YouTube video by the excellent pelvic physiotherapist Carly Wallace (Restore Your Pelvic Floor, @carlywallacepelvichealthph5730) shows it as an entire big, broad sort of *fruit bowl* of muscle, a basin of muscle, inside which (ideally, neatly) sits our bladder, our uterus and our bowel.

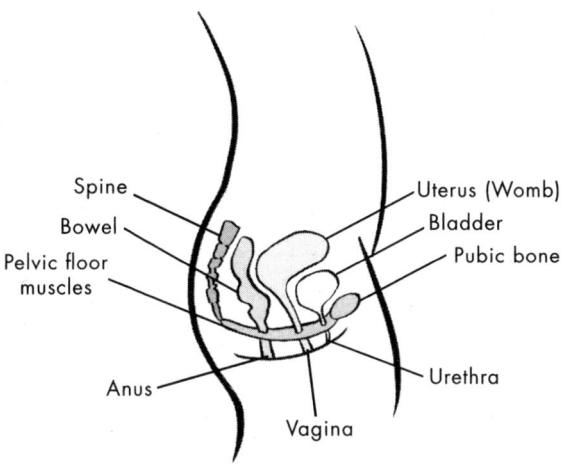

The urethra comes through the muscles at the front; so does the vagina and the anus (rectum, bum, however you know yours). Kegels are a contraction, a squeezing and a lifting, of all those muscles – this, I realise, is where I and many other women before me have gone wrong in our understanding of Kegels. Merely tensing the I-don't-want-to-pee-yet muscles – which is what I'd always done – isn't actually enough to enhance pelvic floor strength. You have to think longer and broader than that: all the way along that cradle, from the muscles at the back of your body, around your bum, through the pee-muscles and up to the front of your lower belly, the pubic bone.

One of my many Pilates teachers tells me to think of the pelvic floor as the clasp along the top of a ziplock freezer bag, and clench as if you're doing up one of those, from one end to the other.

What weakens the pelvic floor? I ask.

"Pregnancy, childbirth and age," Dr Wright says. "It's a double insult to women, I would say. The weakness starts mechanically in pregnancy and childbirth [the pressure of the growing baby, and the force with which it comes out of your body can weaken it], then can get worse, when our oestrogen levels drop, going through the menopause."

It is not therefore, a problem that just affects women who've given birth vaginally – not by any means. It'll come for all of us, to some degree or other, with time.

A weakening pelvic floor is a major issue, not just an embarrassing one. First, because it can mean you lose control of when you pee, which means your lifestyle is massively disrupted, horribly limited; your social life, your work life, your sex life, the whole shebang.

Furthermore, pelvic floors hold the womb, bladder, bowel and cervix up and *in*. If those muscles weaken, there's a chance those organs will fall down and *out*, which is what is meant by the term "prolapse", and which can only be corrected by specialist physiotherapy or surgery – and really? Who wants their inside organs on the outside?

Pelvic floors are crucial to sexual function. A weakened pelvic floor can make sex painful and reduce sensation; a stronger one, I learn from yet another brilliant pelvic floor influencer guru @femalephysioco, will create a stronger orgasm – although equally, too tight a pelvic floor can lead to pelvic pain. They also provide lower-back stability: a weak pelvic floor can contribute to back pain, a strong one will help alleviate it. Indications you may have a weakened pelvic floor include: leaking urine when you sneeze or cough; having to wipe your bum several times after you've had a bowel movement; wind from either your bum or your vagina, particularly when you're doing things like bending forward or lifting something up; tampons which dislodge or fall out; a sensation of bulging in your vagina, or any sensation of heaviness or aching in or around it.

Right, so: how do we strengthen them? Kegels?

"Yes," says Dr Wright.

How can we tell if we're doing it right, though?

"If you put two fingers in the vagina," Dr Wright says, "which physios do – we have specialist pelvic floor physios in this country, but we need to have more. So put two fingers in and squeeze… That's the mechanism by which you strengthen your pelvic floor."

Dr Philippa Kaye suggests imagining you are trying to suck up a piece of popcorn from a chair with your vagina. "Women seem to automatically know what I mean!"

"I'm campaigning to the government to try and make awareness [of pelvic floor strengthening] better," Dr Wright continues. "My old boss used to say, it's like flossing your teeth. As in: it's a pain, it's annoying, you just have to do it every day, but you are then holding off potential problems later in life. Incontinence – and prolapse, which is pretty miserable. They're much better at it in France."

I know this, somehow, God knows how, as I've never given birth at all, let alone in France; but somehow – probably through the gift of vaguely salacious coverage in the press – I do know that, after you give birth, a French midwife will visit you with a box of tricks designed to help restrengthen your pelvic floor, including an electrical device that will contract the muscles surrounding your vagina – Slendertone for the pelvic floor. It's all government mandated, the French call it "*la rééducation périnéale après accouchement"*, or "perineal retraining after child-birth", and while it's inspired some feminist eye-rolling based on the suspicion this is all about becoming adequately… uh, firm, again, for the delectation of *ton mari*, your husband, who might well be tempted to go off and find himself a mistress if you don't, you know how the French are…[34] There's a massive health argument for it, clearly, never mind that this argument does rather assume good sexual function is only important to men, when… Well. It's not, is it?

So when should we start doing all this, caring for our pelvic floor? After we give birth? Mid-30s? 40, max?

"Ideally, at school."

Blimey! Really?

"Yes. Start at school, do them every day, for the whole of your life."

And how would Dr Wright advise we do them?

"I would encourage women to access specialist help. But… obviously, sometimes it's difficult accessing help, medical, physio people. Some women buy things on the internet. You can get cones; you can get bulbs that are supposed to help with your pelvic floor."

When I ask if they actually work, she says that it is still always best to do it under physio guidance, as some devices are too heavy and just drop out.

Yikes.

"That makes your pelvic floor worse. But there are some really

---

34 Off topic but, apparently, despite their reputation, the French aren't more inclined towards infidelity than the British – they're actually less inclined.

good things with bio feedback, a device that goes in your vagina and when you squeeze it, it [syncs with an app on your phone and] tells you how hard you're squeezing, and that makes you more aware of what you need to do." She tells me she herself refers people to Carly Wallace. The NHS Squeezy App is also a valuable resource.

"NHS England has developed some more pelvic floor material. Often women go to all sorts of sources, mainly friends, the internet, which is completely unfiltered. It would be really good to have more accurate sources people can refer to."

It was probably from one of those inaccurate sources that I'd got the idea we can strengthen our pelvic floors by delaying peeing – apparently, this isn't useful.

In the case of a pelvic floor weakened by menopause, when diminishing oestrogen lessens the malleability and flexibility of those muscles, as well as reducing the moisture and overall health of the mucosa, "oestrogen pessaries to the vagina area can help with the vagina, the bladder and the pelvic floor," says Dr Wright.

I ask Dr Wright and Dr Malik what else they'd like us to know about our vaginas. "Vaginal cancer is one of the most important. It's quite rare. But it's something that's notoriously late in diagnosis because women don't notice, or if they do notice, they feel shy talking to their doctor about it," says Dr Wright.

According to recent statistics, one in 1421 British women will be diagnosed with vaginal cancer in their lifetimes, the symptoms of which include: pain in the pelvic area, or rectum (anus, bum); a lump in the vagina; blood in the urine; an increase in the frequency of urination during the day and/or at night; a change in the colour of the urine, darker, or rusty or brown. Also: bloody vaginal discharge unrelated to menstruation, and pain during, or bleeding after, sex.

And in terms of what the experts want us to know about vulvas: "I suppose we should talk about perception," Dr Wright goes on. "I do see quite a lot of girls and women who want to change the appearance of their labia."

Ah… and that's a new development? Relatively?

"Yes. One we assume is related to pornography. I don't think we know. I'm not aware of good research on that. But it didn't used to happen."

What's the timespan on it? When did you see this begin to happen?

"The last 10, 15 years, I think? Which is really sad. I've had at least two patients who've been very angry with me because I turned them away, saying: 'This is the spectrum of normal'. Which is what people need to hear, because it's true. And they've come back saying: 'You weren't sympathetic, and I've found a surgeon who's agreed to do it.'"

As in perform surgery on their labia?

"Yes. People think they look wrong."

There are positive moves forward as well, she says. "People are feeling like they can disclose abuse, now; they feel they can tell someone. And the HPV vaccine."

"The other thing I feel really passionate about," says Dr Malik, "I am a woman of colour. I am of Asian descent. My parents came from Pakistan. The biggest, biggest hole in women's healthcare is ethnic minority women's health. I was on Woman's Hour about a month ago, talking about the latest government survey asking women about their health."

This was a major survey into women's health, announced by the UK government in the autumn of 2023, and launched in 2024. It was controversial because it was only open to women aged between 16 and 55, although that, Dr Malik thinks, is the least of its limitations.

"This is an almost identical survey to the one they did in... I think it was 2021." The UK's 'Women's Health – Let's Talk About It' survey was indeed launched in March 2021.

"And if you look at who answered that survey: white middle-class women in the southeast. No one over 55. Virtually no one of colour. Virtually no one from the north. Virtually no one from a working-class estate, virtually... Actually *no one* who doesn't speak English. Doesn't have the internet. I once did a talk broadcast to the Middle East, about the menopause. Do you know how much flak I got, talking about painful sex in postmenopausal women?"

A lot?

"Yeah. I grew up in Lancashire. Burnley. I went to school in Blackburn. My parents were GPs in Nelson for 30, 40 years, I grew up doing community work with my parents, because there's a massive Asian/Southeast Asian population. My mum is 83 and she still runs a women's health organisation, teaching women English, teaching them about healthcare. You know, I've seen women in labour: I come into an Asian woman's room, and her bottom's not been wiped, her bed's not been changed, because she doesn't speak English. That doesn't happen to them all. But... who's talking about the menopause to Black and Asian women? Who's translating the menopause leaflets and handing them out to my mum's organisation, to give to women in their own language? Who's actually talking to them in their own language? They may not read, some of them. How many women do you know who are Black and Asian, who have painful sex after the menopause, who will go to their GP and talk about it? The government has surveys – but they don't look at who answers it."

Because they don't care?

"I don't think they don't care. Government does care, or it wouldn't try to help people. But it's not effective, I do see that. I'm more interested in how to make it more effective than just whinging about it."

Dr Malik takes a breath.

"I don't know why I'm so worked up about this! I'm getting old!" she says.

I'm glad you are, I say. Someone's gotta.

"We've gone off the vagina," she says.

Yeah, but it's important.

WHAT I KNOW NOW

- The vagina is the channel from the womb to the outside world. Not to be confused with the vulva – the visible outside area of your genitals.

- It is made of mucosa – moist tissue.

- It changes over the course of your life: in puberty, pregnancy and again in menopause.

- It is supported by the pelvic floor – a big bowl of muscles that hold it inside your body, along with your bowel, bladder and womb.

- The pelvic floor gets weak as a result of pregnancy, childbirth and menopause, and it is essential we strengthen it by contracting and releasing it on a daily basis with pelvic floor exercises.

- The clitoris is not just that nobbly tip most people believe it to be. It goes deep into the vulva.

- The vagina is populated by the microbiome, microorganisms essential to its health, and the health of your body overall. You can protect it and prevent yeast infections such as thrush by not wearing pants overnight.

- A healthy vaginal microbiome plays a vital part in protecting women from urinary tract infections, to which we are 30 times more prone than men.

CHAPTER FIVE

HOW BOOBS WORK

I cannot remember growing boobs. I cannot remember getting my first bra. I know it's supposed to be momentous and all – an amazing, awful, enthralling, heady, terrifying expansion of flesh and your understanding of yourself, a foreshadowing of all kinds of horror and glory and worry and sense of identity to come – but I can't.

I *can* remember realising – aged 11 or thereabouts – that my thighs were jiggling and bobbling around under the blue-piped hem on my broderie anglaise ra-ra skirt in a way they never had before, that they were no longer stick thin and contained. I remember not feeling good about that, not at all – actually, I feared it as all girls somehow learn to fear the acquisition of fat – feeling perturbed and powerless in the face of it, understanding on some fundamental level that this was nothing to do with me as a person, nothing to do with the things I wanted for myself, or choices I made, and everything to do with me as a biological creature on a hormonal schedule compelling me towards reproduction at quite an intense speed…

But breasts?

Didn't notice them until they were there. Perhaps because mine didn't develop especially early, or especially late, or especially large. Perhaps my sense of them got lost in the general melee of boob growth going on all around me.

I do remember – aged 16, 17 or so – coming to understand my breasts had a value to me that was complicated and – aged 18, 19, 20 – potentially even fiscal, that I was valued *by* them, *for* them, that I could leverage them for attention and admiration and even cold, hard cash, if I wielded them in the right way, for extra tips, from the business side of the cocktail bar where I worked to fund my first year at university, for example. So began a period of experimentation, and confusion/compromise, feminist-politics-wise. Was it reasonable to leverage my breasts for attention and money, to use the preposterous, questionable hold they had over men, against them? Or was it a sell-out, a leaning-in to the idea they somehow embodied the beginning and end of my worth?

It certainly isn't as if how attractive they make me is the beginning and the end of my relationship with my boobs. I've groaned as they grew pre-menstrual and swollen. I've had them practically ironed flat by mammogram machines. If I can't remember acquiring my first bra, I can certainly remember my quest to find The Perfect Bra, you know the one: as stable as it's pretty as it's washable as it lies discreetly under every single top I own, a quest, I should add, that I'm still on.

I've called them tits and knockers and bazoingas and "the girls" (my country and western phase); but mainly boobs. I've been photographed with them out for club flyers and even for the cover of a high-minded magazine.

If I've never breastfed (no kids), or contemplated altering them surgically, I've watched on and conferred with and supported friends who did. I've also watched, pathetic and hopeless and wondering what I could possibly say to make it even a little bit better, while a friend went through, and ultimately, marvellously, survived breast cancer. I know she won't be the only one. Know it might be me, one day.

Boobs. They are obvious and difficult, compromising and delicious. They're arguably the most physically, emotionally and politically dominant part of the female body; a reductive shorthand for all women that is also a really meaningful, integral part of who we are.

But what are they? And how do they work?

I meet Dr Philippa Kaye, GP, writer, broadcaster, bowel cancer survivor, former sexual health advisor for Ann Summers, and most pertinently in this instance, author of the brilliant *Breasts: An Owner's Guide,* published in 2023. We head for a noisy restaurant in north London. She is 45, brusque, endlessly knowledgeable, a flagrant non-sufferer of fools. I order egg shakshuka; she goes for the vegan lamb kawarma, and that's when she starts telling me about how the clitoris works. I mentioned this in the last chapter, but it's worth taking a detour here to explore what Dr Kaye has to say about the history of the clitoris.

"The anatomy of the clitoris wasn't discovered until the 20th century," she goes on, "which, when you think, in comparison with Leonardo da Vinci, who was doing drawings of anatomical man however long ago... [According to leonardodavinci.net, Da Vinci's *The Vitruvian Man* – that line drawing of a hench chap with flowing locks, limbs at assorted trajectories, and highly visible genitalia – was completed around 1487].

"When a woman says: 'No, a bit left, no, a bit right...' it's not that [the clitoris] is moving. It's that they want the whole of it [stimulated], they want left a bit *and* right a bit, *at the same time.*

And if you pull back the hood and expose the glans [the nobble, the 'nose tip'] that's almost too sensitive, because it's got so many nerve endings. That's why, when you look at a sonic sex toy, it's sending waves down into everywhere, which is why it's easier to orgasm."

Blimey, I say.

"None of this had hit the curriculum when I was in medical school [in the late 90s].. I don't know what it's like now. Wherever you look, from porn to the media, to the conversations I have with patients, the focus is still very much on male pleasure, not female pleasure. Lying back and thinking of England."

Still?

"Yup! Women often think they should just suck it up. There are languages where there is not a word for vulva or vagina. It feels sometimes we are so... *nowhere*. Because, if you can't name it, why would you look after it, let alone get pleasure from it?"

That's rubbish.

"Yeah, but... you are fighting thousands and thousands and thousands of years of women being valued for their ability to bear children, and what they look like, and nothing else. And that takes time. So it's frustrating – but that's OK, it takes time."

We have a moment, a slurp of flat white, a forkful of egg.

Then: to the business of the day!

Boobs, I say. What are they?

"They are mammary glands. They're made of a combination of fat and the mammary glands which produce breast milk. They are mostly held up by skin and some connective tissue called Cooper's ligaments." Cooper's ligaments are fibrous, flexible tissue, which reach from the inner portion of the breast to the pectoral muscles; they're named after Sir Astley Paston Cooper, the baronet, surgeon and anatomist who first identified them in 1840. "They're not really held up by anything else. You would expect them almost to be hanging on a structure – but they're not."

I'll later discover that, as a rough guide, B cup breasts weigh around 0.6 pounds each, C cup: around 1 pound each, D: around 1.5 pounds each, while DD/E cup boobs can weigh anywhere between 1.5 pounds and 3 pounds each.

"So there's the body of the breast, what you might think of as the half round of grapefruit, stuck on." She outlines an invisible, pendulous shape with her hand. "But the breast tissue actually extends up to your collarbone. The tail of Spence…" She traces a hand across the top outer portion of her own breast to indicate a section which, on medical diagrams, looks like a sort of upward-reaching eyeline flick on the main body of the breast, or maybe the point on a teardrop, or of an inverted apostrophe. "This extends up into your armpit. That's why we tell you to examine your breasts all the way up to your collar bone and into your armpit."

Gotcha.

"Within the breast, you have what looks like bunches of grapes – lobules – which make breast milk. They're connected by milk ducts to the nipple. The nipple has lots of little holes in it – it's not one hole. So when the milk comes out, if the baby comes off, or you disconnect from the [breast] pump, it's actually like a water fountain with lots of holes."

Or a shower head?

"Yes. And the areola is the darker bit around it."

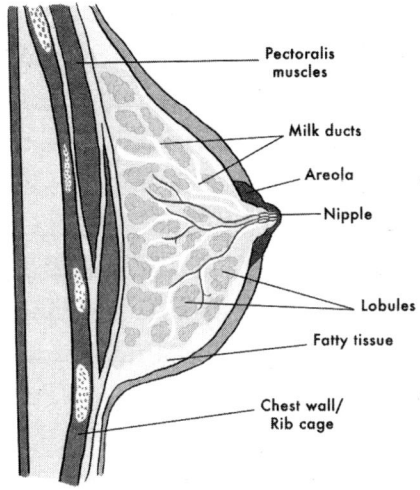

Pectoralis muscles

Milk ducts

Areola

Nipple

Lobules

Fatty tissue

Chest wall/
Rib cage

When do boobs begin to form?

"In the womb. The reason men have nipples is that the bud develops before the Y chromosome turns on testosterone." Until somewhere between five and seven weeks of gestation, the genitalia of all embryos is the same. Then the Y chromosome, which is present in male embryos, kicks in and starts the changes that result in the development of testes. At the same point, five to seven weeks, embryonic girls undergo a thickening in the chest area; this is called the "mammary line", or "milk line". On the outside, though, girls' chests remain flat, indistinguishable from boys', until the very earliest stages of puberty.

I refer back to the Breehl/Caban paper which Dr Charlotte Gribbin printed out for me when I met her to discuss puberty for Chapter 2. It explains that breast development is triggered, along with all puberty, by the hypothalamus, that pea-sized structure located in the depths of the brain, which produces (among other things) gonadotropin-releasing hormone (GnRH), puberty's on-switch.

As we also learned in Chapter 2, the development of boobs in puberty is called "thelarche". At Tanner Stage 2, your nipples become raised, as the increase in GnRH promotes the production of follicle-stimulating hormone (FSH) and luteinising hormone (LH) in the pituitary gland. These hormones whoosh through your bloodstream to your ovaries, which start releasing oestrogen and progesterone for the first time… and, voilà! Breast buds develop: small, hard, flat discs, which raise the breast and nipple. This is Tanner Stage 2, at which the areola, that "darker bit around" the nipple, also starts to increase in size. Tanner Stage 3 sees your boobs continue to grow and develop glandular tissue – the lobes or lobules – the part of the breast that can make milk. In Tanner Stage 4, the areola and nipple (the papilla, the teat, that conical projection in the centre of it all) become raised, standing up and out from the rest of the breast. Tanner Stage 5 is your fully developed "adult" breast, a breast dense with the ducts, tissues and systems ready to make milk should you get pregnant. This typically happens around the age of 17 or 18 but can take until your early 20s.

How big your breasts are is decided by genetics and – to some extent – weight. If you gain weight, your breasts, which are made up of some fatty tissue, may get bigger too; if you lose weight, they might get smaller, though it's not guaranteed.

How do these lumps of tissue, fat, ligaments and so forth come to make breast milk? I ask.

"It's the brain. The brain and the breast together. You get

pregnant. Your levels of progesterone and oestrogen go up during pregnancy, OK? And there are two main hormones involved in the production of breast milk: one is prolactin [produced in the pituitary gland], the other is oxytocin [produced by the hypothalamus, released into your bloodstream by the pituitary]. The level of prolactin begins to rise, but it's only as progesterone begins to fall after childbirth that it's truly unmasked, though some women will produce colostrum during pregnancy." Colostrum, I learn, is the first form of breast milk produced by the body. It's often called "liquid gold" because it's full of nutrients and immune-supporting antibodies for newborns. "Those high levels of prolactin, once unmasked, make the breast produce the milk. As you remove the milk from the breast, you release the hormone in the brain called oxytocin… So the baby goes suckle suckle suckle suckle, and your brain goes, oxytocin: BANG! Then the let-down reflex happens, which makes the milk go to the glands, then come shooting out. You'll feel that as a whooshing sensation. Then, the baby stops going suck-suck-suck-suck, and starts going, more slowly, more rhythmically, gulp, gulp, gulp, gulp. Because now the milk's coming and coming. Once that happens, each time, it tells your brain to produce more, and your breast to produce more. And round and round and round you go."

Is it true that the nutrients in the breast milk vary according to the babies' needs? I ask. Are newborns somehow communicating with their mothers' bodies to influence the very make-up of their milk? Or is that googled-up bullsh*t?

"The nutrients in breast milk vary for lots of different reasons. When it's hot, or at different times of the day, [we] produce different levels of, for example tryptophan." This is an amino acid that also makes us feel sleepy. "So, in an ideal world, you might say: 'If you're expressing at nine o'clock at night, that would be the one that you would give on a night feed, rather than at seven in the morning.' But I say: 'If you're managing to feed your baby: well done!'"

Dr Kaye and I happen to meet during the week the UK releases its national exams, its GCSE results. They, on this occasion, have been accompanied by the results of a University of Oxford study demonstrating that breastfed children were roughly twice as likely to go on to achieve top GCSE results, that their performance in the exams, taken at 16 years of age, improves incrementally the longer the child's mother breastfed them, and that breastfeeding for at least four months significantly increased the likelihood of passing five GCSEs.

"Breast milk is this amazing thing," Dr Kaye continues. "Breastfeeding has health benefits to mum and baby. Yep. And to the child, when they grow up. It is also hard and that difficulty can affect the health of both the child and the mother. So, 'fed is best', *not* 'breastfed is best', in my opinion."

Do breasts do anything for us? For us women, who lug them around for most of our lives? Or are they just there, hanging about and waiting for an opportunity to feed babies?

"It really depends on who's asking. The traditional functions of the breast are not about the woman, no. Women sometimes say breasts are not the bit that belongs to them. They're either to feed an infant, or to attract a man, neither of which are to do with the women themselves. You know, there are studies out there about what men find attractive in female breasts. What size and shape and so on."

Huh? As in: academic studies?

"Yup. Academic studies about breast preference. You've got to wonder how they got the funding… Although there is a value to them, because it changes around the world, and it gives an insight into the social and cultural ideas about what attractiveness is. And that has an importance for society, not because one person should change to be that [ideal], but that different people like different things. For example, they even looked at something as bizarre as, when men were hungry, they preferred women with bigger breasts."

In 2014, Dr Viren Swami of the University of Westminster conducted a study in which 266 men were shown different images of women and asked to rate how attractive they were. The hungrier the men were, the more attracted they were to images of women with bigger breasts. Dr Swami also found, through the same study, that men with a lower socio-economic status preferred larger breasts.

Also:

"There is even research to suggest that men who have very patriarchal, often misogynistic ideas about women prefer a different kind of breast to those who don't," says Dr Kaye. This idea comes from an earlier study by Dr Swami, a 2013 project involving 361 British men, which found that "men's preferences for larger female breasts were significantly associated with a greater tendency to be benevolently sexist, to objectify women, and to be hostile towards women."

How fascinating yet also depressing, I say.

"Well – yes. Where are the studies about what women who

have sex with women prefer? Where are the studies about what women prefer for themselves because they might be thinking about breast pain, or their ability to run for a bus, or their ability to wear a bra or not wear a bra?"

Nowhere?

"Nowhere."

It's beginning to sound like boobs might be more trouble than they're worth, I say. I am unable to find any substantial research at all into how much it costs women to have a pair of breasts over the course of a lifetime – or actually, any research at all. Dr Kaye can think of none. When I google, "How much do breasts cost women?" I'm prompted towards a lot of links to breast aug-mentation services – and one study into the estimated costs of having treatment for breast cancer in Canada (between C$23,275 and C$36,340, or £13,732.50 and £21,436.50). I find a *Daily Mail* article dated 1 May 2009, which suggests the average woman spends £2700 on bras in her lifetime ("but only bothers to wash them SIX times a year")... But what about the cost of breastfeeding? Breast pumps and maternity bras and pads and cloths, and nipple cream? And then, what about how much more women's swimwear seems to cost than men's? What about the financial impact of breast cancer in terms of time off from our careers? And so on and so forth – it really is enough to make me ask: are breasts worth it? Given the cost and the grief, the pain and the obstruction; how self-conscious they can make us feel, how inadequate? How prone to illness they are?

"You've got to wonder if there is gain from having breasts from a sexual perspective, in attracting a mate. There are evolutionary processes, and we think we're not chimpanzees, and we're *not* ...

But we are base on some levels. Our closest animal relative species don't have breasts all their lives. Chimpanzees only develop breasts when they are pregnant and feeding, and then they shrink again."

So why do we keep ours?

"Chimpanzees walk on all fours, mostly, and their genitals are displayed, and when they are ready, ovulating, ready to reproduce, the genitals become very swollen and pink and obvious. There's a big sign: 'Here I am and I'm ready!'. But we stood up. And female genitals are very hidden, which causes all kinds of problems. And so maybe we had to develop breasts to say: 'Here I am, I'm of reproductive age, I'm ready.'"

But we still have them after menopause.

"Yes! You've got to think: why don't they disappear? They change structure after menopause, they become a lot softer. Maybe that's why in some studies, men prefer firmer breasts over softer breasts. Maybe there's some evolutionary thing saying: 'OK a firmer breast is still fertile, while a less firm breast is not.' I don't know. There are still a lot of unknowns."

But basically, what you're telling me is: breasts have no discernible purpose beyond attracting men and feeding babies?

"*No!* They also have a role in pleasure. They're an important part of your arousal. Some women can reach nipple orgasm. Nipple stimulation lights up the same area of the brain as stimulating the genitals. The release of that hormone at breastfeeding – and also at nipple stimulation – oxytocin, that cuddly hormone that helps you bond, that has a role for you as well. So, they are not just someone else's."

Dr Kaye goes on to tell me that seven out of 10 women experience breast pain at some point in their lives. I've certainly had first-hand experience of boobs that felt as if they might burst just before my period, swollen and tender. This, the internet tells me, is related to the ebb and flow of hormones. Increases in oestrogen in the middle of the menstrual cycle cause the breast ducts – which deliver breast milk to the nipples – to enlarge, while an increase in progesterone in the week before your period causes the milk glands – lobules – to swell, both of which can make boobs feel uncomfortable.

On top of that, bigger boobs are cited as a contributing factor in some women's back pain. As my physiotherapist Tom Bradley tells me: "Women with heavier busts often developed them early in teenage years, which means they'll have been teased about it mercilessly by boys and maybe judged on it by other girls and women, so they tend to move into a more protracted position. Think about what you do when you're trying to hide your body: you come forward."

Bradley curves his body protectively in on itself in demonstration.

"That's going to shorten everything on the front side of your body, the abdominals, the pectorals, the front parts of your neck; which means you're much more likely to end up with neck and thoracic spine problems."

Back to Dr Kaye: "The biomechanics is *insane*. And where's the research into that? The research that's been done is on elite athletes. I'm not an elite athlete! Whether or not you can knock off point one of a millisecond off my Personal Best (PB) is irrelevant. And I don't have a PB because I hate running! But where's the research on a normal person? On a pregnant woman? We want pregnant women to exercise during pregnancy – why aren't we looking at the impact of sports bras on pregnancy? If we want women to exercise to stop them having breast cancer – it's one of the things that reduces your risk of breast cancer, and it reduces the risk of recurrence if you've had breast cancer – so where's the study about what happens to your breast and the whole of your trunk if you've had a mastectomy on one side? *Where?* We need more education and help on living with breasts. There isn't much. And when you look at the research into why women give up sport, why girls give up sport, breasts will be there. Not just pain. Embarrassment. You're having mixed sports, as you should, but girls hit puberty before boys, and the comments that come… Why aren't sports bras on the secondary school uniform?"

She is a ferocious advocate for well-fitting bras, which, she says, can help alleviate issues around pain and embarrassment. "They are very helpful. And they're an incredible piece of engineering when they're done properly. By the way, do you know how often you're supposed to change your sports bra?

Once every… three years? Five? Five and half… I have no idea.

"After 25 washes, it begins to change [structurally]."

Nooooooo.

Huge numbers of us are wearing the wrong bra – only one in five of us, 20% of us, is getting it right, according to a study of 41,380 women completed in 2021 by Boux Avenue, a lingerie company which, admittedly, has a vested interest in encouraging us to buy new bras; but, even so, a 2019 *New York Times* article quoted scientists, the shop assistants at Victoria's Secret and even Oprah Winfrey as support (pun, intended) for the same statistic. Dr Kaye's observation of her patients leads her to believe it's a fair estimate.

So pretty much four in every five of us, 80% of us, are not wearing the right bra, which would certainly contribute to our experiencing discomfort and pain, and awkwardness over how we look, and how we – *they* – move.

In addition to which:

"Sizing is so complicated," Dr Kaye says. "There's disparity of sizing in the same companies – a disparity which gets worse the bigger you are; and then the US and Europe have totally different systems again. For example: you know what your band size is?"

I do, I say proudly. 32.

"And your cup?"

D!

"What do you think cup size actually is?"

I motion vague circles around my boobs with both hands.

"Volume?"

Yes!

"It isn't. It's the difference between the band size – the under band – and the biggest part of the breast."

I point at the fullest bit of my breasts, just below the nipples, and she nods.

OK, I say, though I have no real idea how this measurement could help my bras fit, surely a more three-dimensional reference point would be useful?

"I still think it's worth knowing your bra size, as a sort of starting point. Better than going into a bra shop and not having a clue. "But each bra is different so don't get fixated on the size."

Beyond that:

"As a rule of thumb: the bra [back] wants to be parallel all the way round the back. Not a sad face… [an upward-arching frown line described across your back] as lots of people have. And you should be able to get one finger in… [she motions at the front, between the breast bone and central point of the bra, the fabric at the low point in between the cups]… but not more. It should be not so uncomfortable that you can't breathe. So the thing about sports bras: the more constricted they are, the less your breasts will move, but also, you can't breathe, and try exercising if you can't breathe!" You're aiming for a happy-ish medium, a compromise somewhere between the end goal of stable boobs and actually being comfortable enough to train or play your sport. "If you're wearing a sports bra, they're either compression – they literally flatten you – or they are encapsulation: cups. Often, they're a combination. So you want the same thing: not too tight, not too loose. The higher the neckline, the more support it'll give."

I did not know that!

"You want to have adjustable straps. I'm five foot tall, you might be six foot tall," (NB: I'm five foot six inches on a tall day), "but if we've got the same size breasts, you have to be able to adjust the straps," so that they accommodate a bigger or smaller stretch, up and over the shoulders. She says that when you adjust the straps, you should be able to pull them up a couple of centimetres, clear of your shoulders, but not up above your ears, because then, they're going to slip off. If you're bigger-boobed, and you want to avoid them digging in, a wider strap might be better for you.

Also: "You want to fill the cup [with boob], but nothing else should be able to go in there. As my grandmother would say,

'Fold up a tenner so you can get a taxi home', but that's about it. A tenner wouldn't get you very far now." And yet, the bra should be "not so tight that you have a quadruple boob," i.e., not so tight that the flesh visible over the top of the bra, bulges outwards.

"If you have an underwire, the underwire is supposed to follow a specific ligament under the breast. But your ligament and my ligament won't be in the same place. As long as it's not digging into the breast tissue, that's fine. Underwire does give more support."

While we're on the subject:

"There's no evidence that an underwire bra causes cancer. There's no evidence that a black bra can cause cancer. I'm telling you the [unfounded ideas] I've heard. There's no evidence deodorant causes breast cancer."

I'd definitely heard and sort of assimilated the deodorant connection at some point (though also decided I'd take that risk, rather than be sweaty, which has actually worked out for me, now I know there is no evidence of risk at all).

What I did *not* know was that there's a connection between being taller and a higher risk of breast cancer. In an article published in July 2011 by Cancer Research UK, researchers found "a 16% higher relative risk for every extra 10cm (4 inches) of height." They were also, it went on to say, stumped as to why.

Beyond acquiring better-fitting bras, what else helps us look after our breasts and minimise the pain they cause us, the risk of illness?

"The first thing is: breast awareness. You have to know your normal, in all areas of your body. I don't care if its gynae health, discharge health, when you open your bowels, what your breasts are like. You have to know what your normal is. Your breasts will be different to mine. Maybe you have always had inverted nipples. Whatever it is. You have to know your breasts and you have to regularly examine your breasts. Ideally, we like you to examine your breasts after your period because they're less likely to be lumpy; if you are having periods, you should still know what they feel like at different points. So: 'Before my period, this one's always a bit more tender than the other one' – whatever it is. And if you're not having periods, you still need to examine.

How often? Once a week?

"Once a month. Because: one, they change; two, if you're having so much anxiety that all you're doing is checking your boobs all day, you're not living. Once a month. I would say 'Feel on the First' [of the month] is the best way to remember."

The NHS website agrees wholeheartedly on the "know what's normal" approach. It suggests checking your boobs in the shower or bath "by running a soapy hand over each breast" up to the collarbone, referencing the tail of Spence, "and up under each armpit". You should also look straight on at your breasts, in the mirror. You're looking, it continues, for:

- A change in size, outline, or shape of breast.

- A change in the look or feel of the skin on your breast, such as puckering or dimpling, a rash or redness (on darker skin tones redness is harder to see, instead the skin may look darker).

- A new lump, swelling, thickening or bumpy area in one

breast or armpit that was not there before.

- A discharge or fluid from either of your nipples.

- Any change in nipple positioning, such as your nipple being pulled in, or pointing differently.

- A rash (like eczema), crusting, scaly or itchy skin or redness on or around your nipple.

- Any discomfort or pain in one breast, particularly if it's a new pain and does not go away (although pain is only a symptom of breast cancer in rare cases).

In the UK, all women between the age of 50 and 70 are called by the NHS for routine mammograms – an X-ray of the breast, used to detect early signs of breast cancer – every three years. Obviously, you should attend every last one of them. After 70, you are still eligible for these mammograms every three years – you just have to contact your local screening unit.

Finally, I ask Dr Philippa Kaye if there's one thing she wishes more women knew about their boobs – or about health, generally.

"That you don't have to put up with it," she says. "Whatever 'it' is."

You think we should complain more? I ask.

"It's not complaining. It's saying: 'This is what I need.'"

WHAT I KNOW NOW

- Breasts are glands, a combination of fat and mammary tissue, which produce breast milk.

- They begin to exist when a female embryo is between five and seven weeks old. During the pubertal stage known as thelarche, the newly released hormones oestrogen and progesterone cause the formation of breast buds. Through the course of puberty, these become fully developed breasts.

- They're held up by skin and connective tissue called Cooper's ligament. Which isn't much, given that a B cup breast can weigh around 0.6 pounds, a DD or E cup up to three pounds each.

- This means a well-fitting bra is incredibly important – yet 80% of women do not wear the right-sized bra.

- Women spend an average of £2700 on bras in a lifetime.

- The body of the breast contains lobules. These look like bunches of grapes. They're where breast milk is made. They are connected to the nipples by milk ducts.

- Human females are the only species to have breasts at all times. Chimpanzees – our closest animal relative – only develop breasts when they are pregnant and feeding, after which, they shrink again.

- There is a link between being taller and increased rates of breast cancer – though no studies have yet been able to prove what it is or why it seems to happen.

- There's no evidence to support ideas that black bras, underwired bras or deodorant cause breast cancer.

CHAPTER SIX
FERTILITY AND INFERTILITY

I don't have children. This is entirely my choice. I realised, very young, aged literally seven, that I didn't want kids, persisted with that choice through a hundred, thousand, however-many people telling me I was wrong, should change my mind, would live to regret it, would die alone on account of it... and am happy with that decision, far happier than they ever thought I would be, because: guess what? Turns out I knew, better than they, what was right for me, my body, my lifestyle, my future.

However, this does mean I am spectacularly ignorant on the issues of fertility and infertility. My concern was only ever how not to get pregnant. It was never how can I? Or when should I? Or should I, with this person; or should I hold out for someone better? Definitely not what if I can't? Or why can't I? What's wrong with me? What am I, if I can't be a mother? What do I mean?

All around me, friends got pregnant and had babies, struggled to get pregnant, lost pregnancies to miscarriage, persevered with IVF, got pregnant that way, or gave up and grieved. Some froze their eggs, some adopted, I... showed compassion and felt for them, without any real understanding of what was going on, what they were going through. I did get a sense that a lot of my contemporaries seemed to have at least some issue with conceiving, and wondered whether that was that normal, but I certainly didn't stop to think that might be because none of them actively started trying until their early 30s (which seemed absurdly young to me). We gaped and tsked at the audacity of the term "geriatric pregnancy" being applied to those who conceived over the age of 35 (NB: apparently this term is no longer in wide use), until those of my friends who were over 35 and trying to get pregnant began thinking it might not be too wide of the mark ("We are not supposed to be doing this at 40," a friend – pregnant with her first child at 40 – said to me once). But largely, I didn't think about fertility much at all, until I began work on this book.

Here's what I found out, almost immediately, really without having to look very far or hard or even *at all*: our female bodies are at the most fertile when we're in our late teens and 20s. As early as 27, our fertility begins to dwindle. At 32, that dwindling can begin to accelerate; at 35, things can start to get really tough if you're in the conception business. By 40, you've got less than a 5% chance of getting pregnant naturally in any given menstrual cycle. One Norwegian study found that women aged between 25 and 29 have a 10% chance of miscarrying a pregnancy, that this rose rapidly after 30, and by 45, stood at around 53%. We just *are* built to have babies before we're 27, certainly by 30, 31 – yet we're not doing that. We're actually doing the opposite of that, having children later and later all the time. Most women have their first child at 32, according to figures published by the Office of National Statistics in 2024; first-time mothers, the ONS observed, are now 10 years older than those born in 1950, who had their first baby at an average age of 22.

This is a really inconvenient biological truth, right? One that runs in contradiction to both feminist thought and our readiness, emotionally and financially, to have children at the point when our biology is most capable of it. And then, there's how much damage pregnancy in our late 20s, very earliest 30s, does to our professional lives – because those years, when our body is most ready and eager for pregnancy? Those years are also, by hideous coincidence, precisely the ones during which we must work hardest, if we are to establish ourselves in a career context.

And anyway – assuming we somehow overcome all that, the financial, professional and emotional precariousness of being in our 20s – to roll with our ovaries – to have a baby before we're 27: who, exactly, should we be having them *with*? Given that dating-app culture and brutal economic realities seem to have intersected to prevent young men from evolving emotionally or financially to the point where they're able to commit to a second date, let alone, parenthood?

It might also feel as if we're being distracted from this tough truth by news stories about famous, beautiful women, who have babies at 49, 50, 51, older even ("Yeah, but – do you *know* how many of them use egg donors but never quite mention it?" whispers my incorrigible friend, the showbiz reporter); or "female-friendly" employers offering egg freezing as part of their benefits package.

Then – there's all that time spent at school, being told how important it is not to get pregnant, a hangover from the 80s and 90s, when Britain had one of the highest teenage pregnancy rates in Europe.

That last point is something Dame Lesley Regan, professor of obstetrics and gynaecology at Imperial College London and the UK's women's health ambassador, has been seeking to change – at least, balance – for some time.

"We need TikTok videos, don't we?" she said during a 2022 fertility conference. "Remember that your ovaries get worn out or they get tired or they get too old… We've got to impress on [young people] the importance of all of those things and of taking charge of their fertility, either to explore it or to curtail it."

I zoom her.

"Can I put the TikTok quote into context?" says Professor Regan (who is *extremely* direct, *extremely* busy, fresh off a call with Maria Caulfield, previously the Conservative MP for Lewes, a former nurse who, at the time of our call, was serving as parliamentary under-secretary of state for women.)

Of course.

"We were talking about how so many women now have postponed childbearing until much later in their lives, because they are establishing careers. That's also been fuelled by the revolution in reproductive technology – and the ability to have fertility treatments. That's been part of my professional life for a long time, I'm very supportive of all that; but I think it has meant that we've now got a generation of younger women who think that they can turn the clock back on their ovarian function by going to technology. And for many, that is successful, but for some it's a very, very sharp slap in the face, when they find that they can't do it."

Because biologically, our bodies are primed to have children when we're in our late teens and 20s?

"Biologically, the evidence is fertility is at its highest in the 20s, possibly for some women, the early 30s. Age is the immovable factor."

"The biggest single factor is age," agrees Dr Catherine Hill, interim chief executive of the Fertility Network, the British charity that gives support and advice to people dealing with fertility issues. Dr Hill became interested in fertility issues because "I was diagnosed with chlamydia days before my 21st birthday, which was obviously a massive shock. Chlamydia damaged my fallopian tubes, which meant I would need IVF to conceive." Even with IVF, it took Dr Hill five years of treatment to have her daughter.

But it's age, not STIs, which is responsible for most female fertility issues.

"We ran a fertility education campaign a little while ago," Dr Hill tells me. "It was: Every woman should know her fertility vital statistics: 28, 35 and 42. At 28, our fertility has already begun to fall. At 35, female fertility plummets. Age 42, your chances of becoming a biological mother are vanishingly small. And by biological mother, I mean conceiving using your own eggs."

Dr Hill says female fertility reduces over time due to the decrease in the number of eggs – we are, you'll recall, born with all the eggs we'll ever have; we can only lose them over the years – but also due to the quality of those remaining eggs. "There are chromosomal changes, as we get older. So you can have an AMH (anti-Müllerian hormone) test, which is touted as a 'fertility test', but it only gives you information on the number of eggs that you have; it says nothing about their quality. I had an AMH test at the start of my fertility treatments. I was told I had the eggs of a 30-year-old – I was nearly 40. Wonderful. But when I did have fertility treatment, I had multiple miscarriages, because my egg quality at that age wasn't very good."

What do we mean, I ask, by a "good-quality egg"?

"The egg is the largest cell in the body. It has to have no chromosomal damage in order to produce – when combined with a sperm – an embryo that will keep on developing. And if there are chromosomal abnormalities in the egg, then you're not going to get a healthy embryo."

Chromosomal abnormalities are issues at a DNA level – chromosomes are made of protein and a single molecule of DNA.

"By the way, over the age of 40, you'll see a [chromosomal] decline in sperm quality. It doesn't follow the same curve as women's does; it doesn't fall rapidly in the same way. But over the age of 40, there is a decline. Say if you are a young woman with an older man, you are more likely to have miscarriages, because of the sperm quality."

So men are a contributing factor in fertility issues? I ask Dr Hill. I'm slightly furious with myself that it hadn't occurred to me before, that I'd so mindlessly assumed fertility was women's business.

"Oh, yeah! One in six people experiences infertility, according to data from the World Health Authority." WHO figures suggest fertility issues impact 17.5% of the adult population, so yes, roughly one in six, while NICE, the National Institute for Health and Care Excellence, estimates it affects one in seven heterosexual couples in the UK. Dr Hill also cites data from the Human Fertilisation and Embryology Authority (HFEA), the

UK governmental body that monitors fertility treatments. "One of their fertility trend reports from – I think it was 2018, 2019 – had data for the first time which showed that, of all the people seeking fertility treatment at UK fertility clinics, it was more likely for the couple to have a male factor fertility problem than anything else."

Blimey.

"I think [it's] 37% male, 33% female, and the remainder: a mixture of factors and unexplained infertility, because sometimes, you just don't know. But it clearly underlines that fertility is a male issue [as well]." She adds that some andrologists (medical specialists who deal with illnesses which affect men) and urologists (medical experts in the female urinary system and the male genitourinary tract), think the figure is probably higher than that.

It makes me think of a friend whose ex-partner had fertility issues, a situation that eventually broke them up, and who once said to me: "It doesn't even matter if it's them or you. The woman is the one who ends up with her feet in the stirrups, either way."

In a very real and urgent sense… it *does* matter though, Professor Regan points out, because issues with sperm can often be much more easily treated and resolved than those that impact women. "Men make new sperm every 10 to 12 weeks. Many of the factors around morphology – how the sperm look, how they wriggle, the shape – are affected by lifestyle issues." She explains that this is the rationality behind telling men who get a poor sperm count or analysis to wear boxer shorts, rather than tight-fitting underwear, as this can make the testicles overheat and as a result, negatively impact sperm count; to stop cycling, as research has suggested that it can reduce sperm count, motility, concentration and morphology; and to stop drinking and smoking. If you repeat the analysis three months later, you're likely to find that they have a new lot of sperm.

It is clearly of some importance that we recognise fertility to be a male issue, too; and that we destigmatise the investigation and diagnosis of male fertility issues.

But this is, ultimately, a book about female bodies, and so I go on to ask Professor Regan:

Which factors other than age impact fertility in women?

"One: smoking. If you were to smoke a cigarette, within less than a minute, I could identify nicotine derivatives in your follicular fluid, in your ovary. Two: having had a previous successful pregnancy, that is a major predictive factor."

Of your likelihood of having another one?

"Yes. I explain it as, it's a bit like putting on stockings, tights. Once you've put on your tights, they've changed, they've stretched a bit, and they're more able to... cope with things."

What else?

"Obesity is a major factor. Society doesn't like engaging with it."

Yes, Dr Hill mentioned it too; and NHS guidance on IVF is that you must have maintained a BMI of between 19 and 30 (even as low as 25, in some trusts), for six months before seeking treatment, to qualify for it for free.

But why does obesity negatively impact our chances of getting pregnant?

"It's a big, big problem," Professor Regan says. "People get really cross with you [if you raise it]... but you've got to persuade women that fat is not padding. It's an organ in its own right. When you have too much fat, this organ starts producing inflammatory chemicals called cytokines, and that can affect the metabolism of the ovary. And it can also affect the ability of the tiny, fertilised egg, the tiny embryo, to embed successfully into the womb lining. For women who are having fertility treatment because they're not ovulating, the drugs that you use to make them ovulate do not work as well [if they have a high BMI]. Look: that doesn't mean that every fat woman has this problem. But if you're overweight, you're obese, and you come with a history of miscarriage or of infertility, the first thing to do is to shed the weight, because that is going to definitely affect the way your ovary metabolises. Being very underweight does as well, which is a very important thing; it's not just the fat – it's the lack of weight as well. They are a much smaller group of women, but it's remarkable. And if you have women who've got polycystic ovaries, and infertility and irregular periods or absent periods, and have got a high BMI – you get their BMI down to 30, and they often start menstruating and ovulating spontaneously."

EGG FREEZING

What, then, are we to do about our fertility, if our biology means we should be having babies at 27, but our entire world – our work life, our financial status, our relationship status and our emotional state – makes that impossible?

I know that egg freezing is often perceived as, if not The Answer, then certainly An Option. This process involves extracting a woman's eggs when she, and they, are young, cooling them and storing them in tanks of liquid nitrogen so that, even as she ages, they do not. They can then theoretically be defrosted and used in a pregnancy later in life, when she, or her career, or her partner, are finally ready. The services that offer it talk about it in terms of "elective fertility preservation", and employers who would like to be perceived as progressive and female friendly make a big, public deal about how they will pay for female staff to freeze their eggs, as part of their benefits package (Google and Bumble among them). Egg freezing was also one of the products I noticed being forcefully marketed at commuters from billboards on a Tube wall.

I call Sophia Money-Coutts, to see what she thinks. She's a journalist and author who's written extensively about her decision to freeze her eggs; in 2020, she wrote and presented a podcast called Freezing Time, on the same subject.

She and I meet for coffee and toast on the morning the HFEA releases figures that show a dramatic increase in British women freezing their eggs, a 64% rise: 4215 cycles in 2021, up from 2576 in 2019.

"It's Covid," says Money-Coutts.

You reckon?

"Absolutely. Women feel like they lost time."

Money-Coutts got her eggs frozen in 2020, when she was 35. Because of lockdown? I ask.

"No. I'd been thinking about it for about a year and a half. It took me that long to get my head round it. That's the tricky bit. Getting your head round it."

Why?

"Because you're getting your head round how you, a woman in your 30s, are not where you thought you might be. That, and the expense." The process of collecting and freezing eggs in the UK is estimated to cost around £3350, on top of which comes the price of medication required to facilitate collection, which can be a further £1500; *then*, there's the storage fee for the frozen eggs, which can be anything from £125 to £350 a year. Money-Coutts (who is not rich, despite her utterly fabulous name) estimates she spent about £5000 overall on the process.

"Then, there's: 'sh*t! Do I want to put my body through this fairly horrendous process where I'm having to inject it with hormones?', *and* you don't know how many rounds you're going to have to go through either."

So it's an emotional, financial and physical reckoning?

"Yes! And for a lot of people – I didn't have this, but some people do – they don't want to tell their families, or anyone, about it, because there's a lot of shame around it. People are embarrassed. The reason I decided to make the podcast was, about a year and a half before the pandemic, a really good friend of mine started the process of egg freezing. Towards the end of her round, she said: 'Soph, do you mind taking me to the hospital, then coming to collect me, because I'm having my eggs collected?' She was so embarrassed she hadn't told her parents. Not even her mum."

Money-Coutts hadn't always wanted kids, by any means. "No! And I spent my teenage years, like everybody at school, being told: 'Don't get pregnant! Just don't get pregnant!' We had this notion – you know, boarding school – that if we even looked at a man, we'd get pregnant. And then it's confusing, because you get to 30, to the tipping 30 mark, and… I suddenly started noticing all the *Daily Mail* headlines, saying: 'That extra glass of wine is going to make you infertile!' So then it's: 'Hang on, I was being told *not* to do it; now, I'm being told definitely do it! Do it *now*!' You get whiplash. I don't have a biological clock. Never have had. But I decided egg freezing would be a sensible thing to do."

She took 18 months to make up her mind, but also to research. "I did so much research. All the clinics have open evenings you can go to." She eventually settled on the Lister in central London, "went to an open evening with this great doctor, Dr James, lovely and incredibly handsome. I did actually think: 'Can I go on a date with my fertility doctor?'"

That's a topic for another book. In terms of the egg freezing, what happened first?

"I think what every woman then has to go through, is a 'fertility MOT'. I hate the terminology, but there it is, most people call it a 'fertility MOT'."

And what is it?

"You get your AMH check, your anti-Müllerian hormone…" This is the one to which Dr Hill referred, the one that provides a sense of how many eggs you have in your ovarian reserve but which cannot tell you how good they are, or how quickly and easily you will conceive with them. It's done with a blood test, and recommended as a rough, informal guide in helping you more fully understand your fertility. After this, Money-Coutts tells me, you have a gynaecological scan, which looks at your ovaries and your follicles, and in combination with the AMH check, enables the clinic to give you a ballpark figure of the number of eggs you have.

"Based on my MOT, I was looking at [collecting] between 12 and 15 eggs [following one round of hormone treatment]. That's quite a difficult one, because it's an OK number, but they really recommend you get 20 to have a good chance of one 'live birth'. Another phrase I hate, 'live birth.'"

Money-Coutts began taking hormones, "every day for two and a half weeks." Injecting? "Yes."

Was that awful? It sounds awful.

"No! So I started by sniffing a hormone, which basically puts your body in a kind of temporary menopause, stops you releasing eggs, so they don't start ripening [too early]. Did that for about a week, I think, then I started self-injecting, which, before the first one, is terrifying, but when you do it, it's actually really satisfying."

What are you injecting?

"Two hormones."

These are high doses of FSH, follicle-stimulating hormone and LH, luteinising hormone, which are designed to stimulate the growth and development of multiple eggs within your ovaries, all at once.

"I did the injections for about 10 days, then you do what's called a trigger injection, which tells your ovaries: it's time, ovaries! And the ovaries let 'em all out!" The trigger injection is actually a further shot of hormone, which acts as a final push on the maturation of the eggs, and is typically administered 36 hours before the retrieval operation.

Did the hormones impact her emotionally? Physically? I've got one mate who says hers sent her half mad, another (also a writer) who said they made her suddenly incredibly productive, she was up all night, churning out manuscripts…

"I was completely fine. A bit like a Michelin man, I was slowly swelling up. The day before the operation, I remember drifting around my sister's house – I was living there – in my dressing gown, feeling quite gross. Not teary, not emotional. There was one moment when I couldn't get the needle into my belly. That was quite depressing, I was crying then. Because it feels quite lonely at that stage. Actually, it was a week after [the egg retrieval surgery], that I felt most sh*t. Because I think, you've flooded your body with hormones, and now, they're ebbing away. And because of this thing, which women who've gone through egg freezing are at risk of, called OHSS." OHSS is ovarian hyperstimulation syndrome, which causes your ovaries to swell and leak fluid into your abdomen. It can be incredibly painful, and potentially even dangerous. Any woman who undergoes ovarian stimulation for fertility treatments can be at risk. Money-Coutts did not have OHSS, but, of course, became anxious that she might.

And how was the egg retrieval operation? I ask. Do they put you right out?

"No, which is a shame, I love having general anaesthetic."

Me too!

"They used to do general anaesthetic, but since the pandemic, they do what they call 'heavy sedation'. I remember saying to Dr James: 'How heavy?' Because they push a needle through your vagina and into your ovaries. I was like: 'I need sedation'. But I was under for 20 minutes. Really quick."

And you know nothing about it?

"No. Apart from recovery, the swelling and lying on my mum's sofa... But the actual operation? Nothing. Didn't feel anything. Then: no stitches, nothing. In the end, you come round, and all you want to know is: 'How many? How many eggs?' The doctor came into my room and said: 'We got 29; 22, mature – 22 to go in the freezer.'"

So more than you'd expected – more than the magic desirable number of 20?

"Yes. I was really lucky. I've got another friend, she only got one or two eggs. It's really hard when you wake up and the doctor says: 'Sorry, we've only got one or two eggs,' and you've been through all that."

And where, now, are those eggs?

"They've rushed them all from the operating theatre into a lab, where a lab technician looks at them through a microscope and goes: yes, no, yes, no…"

What are they looking for?

"That the eggs are mature enough, so that, when they're defrosted, there's a chance they can be fertilised. There's a big debate about whether it's better to freeze embryos [eggs already fertilised by sperm] than eggs … I asked Dr James about this relentlessly. There is a theory that, if you fertilise an embryo and then freeze it, it is a more stable unit… Apparently, eggs can get screwed up when you defrost them, because they've got quite a high water content, and that water crystallises; but if you freeze embryos, there's less water, therefore less chance to be destabilised when you defrost them."

Money-Coutts decided against freezing embryos, however, not only due to the additional cost (she says it can be around £10,000), but also because you'd also have to pick, and pay for the sperm (possibly another £1500). "It's just another emotional and financial burden," she says.

We are meeting three years on from her retrieval process. Money-Coutts is 38 now, and she has just got her latest bill for egg storage. "Every year, it rolls around: £350." Where actually are they? "In the Lister still, in R2D2-shape cannisters. Mini freezers, in this room, which I'd expected to look incredibly high tech, but it was clearly an old meeting room with all the folders cleared out. They're put in these freezers, with backup generators. It felt fine to see them. Weirdly normal. Quite satisfying, like: great. That is done."

Insurance policy: activated?

"No, no. We have to be careful when you talk about 'insurance policy' because there is no guarantee. I've got 22 eggs, but none of them may work. I interviewed two women on the podcast who also had that amount of eggs, and they didn't have babies from them. I say this again and again: it's no insurance policy."

It should absolutely be said that few eggs frozen are ever even defrosted, let alone used as the basis for a future "live birth". According to an American study published in 2022, the overall chance of a live birth resulting from eggs frozen by a woman aged 38.3 (the average age of women choosing to freeze their eggs), waiting (the average) four years to thaw and fertilise those eggs, was 39%. This rose to 51%, if the woman was younger than 38 when she froze her eggs, and 70% if she was younger than 38 and, like Money-Coutts, thawed 20 or more eggs.

"Women are overly optimistic" about their chances to have a baby when they freeze their eggs, said Dr Marcelle Cedars, professor and director of the division of reproductive endocrinology at the University of California San Francisco, on the study's publication. "The pregnancy rate is not as good as I think a lot of women think it will be. I always tell patients: 'There's not a baby in the freezer. There's a chance to get pregnant.'"

"The stats are really bad," says Money-Coutts. "There is very little data because it's still relatively new, and a lot of the women who've had them frozen haven't come back to use them." According to a recent study led by the Universitair Ziekenhuis Brussel, less than a third of women who freeze their eggs return to use them, and of those that do, only half end up using those frozen eggs in their treatment.[35]

Regarding the data that does exist on pregnancies resulting from defrosted eggs, Money-Coutts tells me that they're "lumping it together, whether you froze your eggs at 30 or 40. You're comparing 30-year-old eggs with 40-year-old eggs? I interviewed one doctor who said he thinks it should happen to every girl on her 21st birthday."

I ask her what her plan is. Has she imposed deadlines on herself? Is there a point where you go: I must thaw my eggs now, and use them, or chuck them out and stop paying the fees?

"When I did it, I remember thinking, 'if I get to 39 and I'm still single, maybe I'll try and have a baby by myself.'"

I ask her if this is still the case.

"I couldn't feel less inclined. I mean, if I met someone and fell in love tomorrow, maybe. But I've got no biological clock. The other thing that's happened in the law, which is useful, is there used to be 10-year limit but the government has changed that, after a lot of campaigning." In 2021, then Health Secretary Sajid Javid announced that storage limits on eggs, sperm and embryos would rise from 10 to 55 years. "So now, if you're 30, it's way more viable, because you don't have to think: 'But when I'm 40, they're all going to be chucked out.'"

So is Money-Coutts just taking every year as it comes? Pay that invoice, see what's what in another year?

---

35 Few women return to their frozen eggs, European study suggests, Human Fertilisation & Embryology Authority, 2021 – https://www.hfea.gov.uk/about-us/news-and-press-releases/2023/few-women-return-to-their-frozen-eggs-european-study-suggests/

"Pretty much. I mean, I do think: would I give them away, if I don't use them? I feel a bit weird about the idea of my genetic children running around without me. I wouldn't have an issue donating them to medical research. But I don't think I could give them to anyone else. Unless I did have children of my own? Then, perhaps. But otherwise: that makes me really sad, the thought of half of me, running around, that I don't know about."

(At the time of publication, Sophia Money-Coutts hadn't yet had a baby – but she had acquired a dog.)

IVF, IUI AND OTHER FERTILITY TREATMENTS

I'm supposed to meet Dr Shazia Malik to talk through IVF – what it means, how it happens, and what it's like to perform it as a doctor – early one Tuesday morning, but she pushes our appointment by a week, because one of her patients goes into labour, which is an even better excuse than Maisie Hill's late-running horse-riding lesson.

Did it go OK? I ask, when we eventually do meet up, for coffee and nice cake.

"Yes!" she says. She beams.

Reproductive medicine is her sub-speciality; something, she says, she was drawn to because: "It's a really broad umbrella... and it allows me to use lots of different skills and bring them together to try and help women with whatever issues they may come with. That's the beauty of it."

What do we mean by "infertility"? I ask.

"It means different things to different people. So I think infertility means that you've been trying to make a baby, and for whatever reason – and there are a multitude of reasons – you, either on your own or with a partner, if you have a partner, have been unsuccessful in that journey. And it means different things to the NHS, it means different things to women of different ages. And it means different things to couples. I think you should define what it means to *you*. But you need to be conscious of the fact that you may not get medical help or even investigation unless you fulfil what either the doctors or the government deem to be something which warrants investigation or treatment."

NICE's current recommendations to the NHS are that women should be considered eligible for three free cycles of IVF if they're younger than 40 and have been trying to get pregnant with regular unprotected sex for two years; or if they haven't become pregnant following 12 cycles of artificial insemination, at least six of which should involve IUI, intrauterine insemination; a process I'll explain shortly.

Women aged between 40 and 42 should be offered one free cycle of IVF if they've been trying to get pregnant through regular, unprotected sex for two years, or they've had 12 unsuccessful cycles of artificial insemination, at least six of which should involve IUI; but only if they've never had IVF treatment before, if they show no evidence of low ovarian reserve, or of poor quality eggs, and if they're fully aware of the additional implications of IVF and pregnancy at this age. Women over the age of 43 are ineligible for IVF on the NHS. Additionally, as Dr Hill and Professor Regan both referenced, NICE's guidelines insist women of any age do not have children already, from either current or former relationships, do not smoke and be of a healthy weight. These are guidelines, however, and not all integrated care, ICBs, the organisations responsible for managing health services in a local population, adhere exactly to them: some ICBs, for example, offer no IVF to women over the age of 35.

"Did you know the thyroid can affect your chances of getting pregnant and miscarrying?" Dr Malik asks me.

I did not. But – *why?* The thyroid doesn't produce sex hormones, does it? And it's in your neck; nowhere near the business end, nowhere near your ovaries, cervix, vagina…

"Because your hormonal balance, your hormonal health, your fertility, is intimately linked to *all* your endocrine organs, of which, one is the thyroid." According to the Mayo Clinic, hypothyroidism, or an underactive thyroid, means your body can't make enough important hormones. Low thyroid levels can affect the release of an egg from the ovary, which can make it harder to get pregnant. Also, some causes of hypothyroidism, like autoimmune or pituitary problems, can affect fertility.

This thyroid connection may also be one of the reasons stress impacts your fertility. As Dr Malik says, "The number of women you'll see, who had a really stressful life event and their periods stopped for six months, a year… Stress can bring forward menopause. Not massively, but it can have an impact."

Is that all about cortisol? The stress hormone?

"Not just cortisol. It's the balance of your hormones. What did I see in lockdown? Women started running, they lost weight. And what did they come to me with? No periods. And that's because your hypothalamus and your pituitary form an axis with your ovaries." She's referring to the way your hypothalamus and pituitary glands talk to your ovaries, tell them to produce oestrogen. "When you run a lot, you switch off that axis," that line of communication. "Oestrogen levels drop. Your period stops."

Is that because, on a primal level, your body thinks you're running from danger therefore you're in no position to get pregnant and give birth?

"Ha. Don't know. You'd have to ask an anthropologist. It's definitely because you lose weight." It is a combination, I discover, of low body fat and being in calorie deficit – burning more calories through exercise than you're consuming. Overexercising itself can disrupt hormones, and then there's the emotional and physical stress it causes.

Which all means that: "If you're underweight or overweight," says Dr Malik, "your chance of being subfertile increases significantly for different reasons."

Professor Regan told me about fat being not padding, but an organ in its own right.

"Yes. Fat stores different hormones; but being very overweight also affects the kind of birth you might have and means you're more likely to have diabetes in pregnancy. Being underweight or overweight means you won't ovulate as regularly, which won't help your chances of making a baby."

In the year after I speak to Professor Regan, Dr Malik and Dr Hill, a revolution happens in the weight loss market. Weight loss jabs like Ozempic and Wegovy become extremely popular. These medications work by mimicking the satiety hormone, GLP-1, which is released by our gut after we've eaten and tells our brain we're full and don't need to eat any more. These jabs convince our brain we're always full, so we eat much less and, as a consequence, lose weight. The ethics, safety, effectiveness and cost of such drugs is heavily disputed at the time of publication; but one unexpected consequence has been "Ozempic pregnancies", women who'd previously had fertility issues becoming unexpectedly pregnant while taking a weight loss medication. This is presumed to be a function of weight loss; though the US Food and Drug Administration advises women to stop taking Ozempic at least two months before a planned pregnancy.

I tell Dr Malik that Dr Catherine Hill had talked about a recent survey that found that "most people going into fertility treatment are experiencing depression, even say they feel suicidal," and that this is the case not just for women, but for men, too. Is that Dr Malik's experience?

"Nobody knows the real figure. But this is why I think there should be mandatory counselling for every part of fertility treatment. All of it. If you go for a fertility check, if you go to talk about freezing your eggs: all of it. If somebody comes to me for a fertility check-up, I say: 'Listen, it's really easy for me to help you do this. But what if I tell you that actually, your egg store is not good? What's your next step? Are you going to have IVF? What do you feel about IVF? Can you afford to have IVF? Because if your results are really not good, you may not fulfil the NHS's criteria. What does your partner feel about IVF? Where's your relationship at?' Because it's easy as doctors to do the tests, or do the treatment…"

But not to necessarily provide emotional support or perspective on next steps?

"Right."

Right. So: IVF. I know it's really expensive, mainly because I'm forever reading newspaper articles with headings like: "I spent £50k on IVF and I still don't have a baby". A friend of mine, pregnant in her mid-40s for the second time (she had her first through IVF at 42), has spent over 100 grand on IVF for this baby (and has endured two miscarriages – one quite late term.)

The HFEA explains that private clinics set their own charges, and that these vary dramatically. The NHS website says, sweepingly, that it may "cost up to £5000 (per cycle, per 'go') or more", but elsewhere, I see figures which vary from £7000 to £17,500. The HFEA points out that different clinics will have different definitions on what a "cycle" even is.

For example: "In some areas one cycle means you get one fresh embryo transferred to the womb and if you have additional, good-quality embryos these can be frozen and one, two or more frozen embryos can be transferred to your womb later on. In other parts of the country, one cycle means you only get one fresh embryo transferred to the womb and no frozen transfers. This means if you wanted to freeze additional high-quality embryos and use them later on, you would need to pay for this." Some clinics, the HFEA continues, will quote costs which cover the treatment itself, and the treatment only – not the very expensive fertility drugs you will need to take to prepare your body for that treatment. It's a minefield; fortunately, the HFEA offers comprehensive guides on how you should choose a clinic.

So, I know IVF is expensive. I also know it's emotionally draining, depression-inducing; that it can even make people contemplate suicide.

But I don't actually know what it is.

Could Dr Malik give me an IVF for beginners course?

"Do you know what it stands for?"

In vitro fertilisation?

"Yes. 'In vitro' means, it's in the lab. Or, in a dish. And we're fertilising an egg. But there are lots of fertility treatments, and they're not all IVF. You can, for example, just do insemination of sperm."

What does that mean? You manoeuvre the sperm into the fallopian tube?

"No. Into the cervix, where it can then swim up to where it needs to be."

This, then, is IUI, intrauterine insemination, "a fertility treatment that involves directly inserting sperm into a woman's womb," according to the NHS' website; it's also the treatment the same site invokes when describing the criteria according to which a woman is eligible for IVF, as discussed above.

So, with IUI, you're kinda giving the sperm an initial boost?

"Exactly. The lab will spin the sperm [sample] and take the best ones, the ones that look normal, are swimming the best, and have the best chance of fertilising an egg." To inseminate the patient, the doctor opens the vagina with a speculum, which allows them to see into it, and then inserts the sperm using a quill, as close to the cervix as possible. The other alternative is to have IVF.

The whole shebang. Tell me about that.

"You have injections, which stimulate your ovaries into producing a lot more eggs than they normally would in one particular cycle." These are the same injections Money-Coutts described in her egg-freezing process; if, in a natural menstrual cycle, we release one, maybe two eggs, with these FSH injections, you'll ideally release considerably more. Those eggs are, as with egg freezing, matured through a further injection, before being collected using a needle passed through your vagina and into each ovary under ultrasound guidance.

"Occasionally," says Dr Malik, "it will have to be done as a laparoscopic abdominal procedure [keyhole surgery], because your ovaries are stuck." In all circumstances, you'll be under sedation or general anaesthetic while this happens.

Then what?

"You collect the eggs. The embryologist will then examine those eggs under the microscope. And then you will have IVF."

Go on...

"IVF can take the form of either just mixing the eggs with sperm, then... seeing; or, it can be taking one sperm and injecting it into one egg. This is called ICSI: intracytoplasmic sperm injection. ICSI is a procedure that happens in the lab; it doesn't affect you, or the person giving the sperm, which may or may not be your partner. It may be a sperm donor."

And why would you do it that way? With ICSI?

"You may do it, because there's not enough sperm. Or, if you're defrosting eggs, frozen eggs, for example. We know ICSI probably increases success rates of IVF."

And that's how you make embryos?

"Yes."

According to the NHS, those fertilised embryos will continue to grow in their lab for up to six days, at which point, the best of them will be selected for a "transfer", to be reinserted into the woman's body.

With what... tool? I ask Dr Malik, who laughs.

"First of all, it's got to be a sterile environment. So – you have your legs up, you have the speculum, then your embryologist will give the embryo to the doctor who's going to do your embryo transfer. There's a tube that goes through the cervix and is very carefully put into the uterine cavity. It's all done under ultrasound control. And also on a screen: you're watching your embryo being transferred."

Wow. How long does that take?

"Seconds. But the reason it takes seconds is that it's a very carefully planned procedure. In the cycle before you have your IVF, you will have had ultrasound scans to check your anatomy, you will have had a little rubber tube put through the cervix into the womb, to check that there are no polyps or anything in the womb lining that would affect implantation of your embryo. In a good clinic, you will have had a dummy embryo transfer. That's so we can check if your cervix is too tight, we can see which way your uterus goes, we can see whether your cervix needs dilating before the embryo transplant. The smoother the embryo transfer, the higher the chance of you being pregnant with it."

I forget to ask Dr Malik if transfer hurts. I google it later and find testimonies explaining that it doesn't particularly; describing it as, at worst, involving some mild cramping. I double-check with my mate P, who had her four-year-old son by sperm donor and IVF.

"Oh, it hurts," she says. How much? I ask. "Well, maybe I'm just one of those women who doesn't like being cranked open with a speculum," she replies. I'm one of those, too, I say. "It hurts like being cranked open with a speculum hurts," P says. Gotcha. "It is over quickly, though," she qualifies.

After transfer, how long does it take the embryo to implant? I ask Dr Malik.

"You're going to do a pregnancy test two weeks later: but it should be implanting before then."

"This is why the womb lining is such an important part of IVF. It's not just about having great embryos. It's like – the soil. You've got this seed... but the soil has to be there."

"There's a whole science behind implantation, behind implantation failure: women who are producing apparently amazing embryos, their womb linings look normal, but they're still not getting pregnant. Why? Implantation."

Does anything help with implantation?

"Reducing stress. Did you know that acupuncture around the time of embryo transfer may increase implantation rates?" I discover that this is also because acupuncture can boost blood flow to the reproductive organs. "I'm forever sending my patients to their local Chinese [practitioners]. They're doctors. They may not speak much English, but they've been doing this for 30 years, like me. Don't take any herbs, because you don't know what's in them and they may affect your IVF."

But: let them stick the needles in?

"Yes! Reduce the stress! Give yourself all the chances!"

But it's not, she tells me, just about reducing stress. Dr Malik says other lifestyle changes can positively impact fertility. Among them, getting enough sleep, quitting smoking and drinking, eating a healthy diet with plenty of antioxidants, cutting back on microplastics by filtering tap water, eating organic food where possible, and not microwaving food in plastic containers, and finding a good balance with exercise and weight.

I have several friends who had babies by IVF, some late in the day, with partners, some on their own, via sperm donor, some who'd started earlyish, and struggled and struggled then just hit on the one clinic, the one doctor, who made it semi-miraculously happen for them. But I also have friends for whom it didn't work out. Who tried and tried and tried, who got into terrible debt for it, who filled themselves with hormones and submitted their bodies to the stirrups and their cervices to the quill and... it never took. They all felt miserable, depressed, as if they'd failed, more than one found their relationships couldn't survive the terrible grief of it; they all, also, felt somewhat cheated by the fertility industry, felt they'd been sold a lie – not necessarily by the clinics and medics, but by the fertility narrative, which tends to be so uniquely focussed on the success stories, the precious, blanket-swaddled, pink-cheeked bundles of joy snatched at the last minute from the jaws of a bleak, empty childless future, like Indiana Jones's hat from under the closing door on a tomb.

So how often does IVF actually work?

According to the HFEA, "Average IVF pregnancy rates using fresh embryo transfers for patients aged 18–34 were 41% per embryo transferred, compared to 6% for patients aged 43–50 when using their own eggs in 2021." The NHS website – where data ends at women aged 42, that's the cut-off point for the NHS's provision of free IVF, as we've noted – has it at: "32% for women under 35. 25% for women aged 35 to 37. 19% for women aged 38 to 39. 11% for women aged 40 to 42."

Which means that, among relatively young women, IVF doesn't work most of the time, doesn't even offer a 50% rate of efficacity.

Beyond that, I wonder, what are the risks of IVF? Other than it not working?

"Taking it from the beginning of the procedure," says Professor Regan, "you can get ovarian hyperstimulation syndrome, which is life threatening." OHSS, which Money-Coutts worried she might be experiencing after her egg collection: though she wasn't. "That's when the ovaries blow up, get very, very enlarged, it can be very, very scary. That's why [for] women with polycystic ovaries, you hope the clinicians looking after them are very conservative about the way they start the stimulation, until they've seen how somebody responds."

Are there issues further into the process? I ask Professor Regan. "If you don't subscribe to a transfer-one-embryo policy [the HFEA recommends what's called 'eSET', elective single-embryo transfers], then you will have a high rate of multiple pregnancies, not just twins, but higher-order multiple pregnancies, and they are all much more likely to result in a neonatal death or a stillbirth, a miscarriage or a pregnancy with maternal complications such as high blood pressure, diabetes, etc. I mean, as a mother of twins, I know how scared I was thinking, 'Oh my God, how did this possibly happen?' I didn't have fertility treatment. But it was very, very scary, because I was just so aware of all the awful complications I could have. Of course, some twin pregnancies are actually fine, but they are definitely a risk factor. And there's all sorts of evidence demonstrating that other complications, medical complications, can be increased in a woman with previous infertility, who goes through IVF. Hypertensive disorder [high blood pressure] … things like that. And remember, it's not an even playing field: the vast majority of women you have in fertility treatment are a bit older, so they've got a greater risk of having maternal diseases anyway, increasing in prevalence as decades go past, compared to a 25-year-old."

None of which is to say: Women, abandon your career prospects and have your kids at 25! Before it's too late and you suddenly find yourself, aged 45, giving all your money and your mind to an IVF process that doesn't work a lot of the time and might rob you of your savings, and your relationship, while exacerbating your high blood pressure and your anxiety. Because IVF clearly does work sometimes, and any medicine that contributes to freeing women up, at least a bit, has got to be a good thing, hasn't it? On which, in the summer of 2024, early results of a long-term study into the possible repurposing of an immunosuppressant called rapamycin suggested that it could be a safe way of delaying the menopause by up to five years. The drug, currently prescribed to organ transplant patients, appears to delay the ageing of ovaries by 20%. Which is exciting. And there will, presumably, be more medical developments of this kind.

The problem is, I guess, that we can't entirely rely on it. On any of it. On rapamycin or egg freezing or IUI or IVF or whatever comes next.

All we can do is *know this*. Understand it. Factor it in. Teach it, in schools, to boys, as well as girls, and in life, to all the men who are no longer in school. Let them know your biology's on a schedule – and furthermore: so's theirs. They might fancy themselves a starter version of all those octogenarian rock and movie stars who somehow get their 30-year-old girlfriends up the duff in between world tours, but a) those octogenarian rock 'n' movie stars are, in all likelihood, quietly taking advantage of fertility treatments, and b) there's only one Mick Jagger, anyway.

Until we get a fundamental restructuring of society overall, until we start properly supporting young women out of the workplace to have children, then back into it, once they're ready to pick up their careers where they left them off, until we make childcare affordable... equipping ourselves with knowledge of how our fertility operates, what helps it, and what gets in its way, is pretty much all we've got.

WHAT I KNOW NOW

- Age has the greatest impact on female fertility, because it means a decrease in both the number of our available eggs and their quality.

- Our fertility can begin to decrease as early as 27; by 32, it's definitely on the slide.

- At 35, our fertility begins to decrease more rapidly. At 40, we have a less than 5% chance of getting pregnant in one menstrual cycle.

- Sperm is also subject to the ageing process. As eggs decline on a chromosomal level with age, so does sperm.

- Male fertility issues – low-quality sperm – often play a role in difficulties conceiving. They're also relatively easily rectified with better lifestyle choices, because men create a new batch of sperm every 10–12 weeks. By giving up smoking and drinking, wearing less tight underwear and cycling less, men can improve their own fertility.

- Smoking, obesity and being underweight all affect a woman's chances of conceiving, as do thyroid issues, and stress.

- The popularity of egg freezing among 30-something women is increasingly rapidly. According to the latest available figures from the HFEA, the Human Fertilisation and Embryology Authority, egg freezing and egg storage increased from 2576 cycles in 2019 to 4215 in 2021 (a 64% rise).

- Less than a third of women who freeze their eggs return to use them, and less than half of those will end up using those eggs in treatment.

- IVF stands for "in vitro fertilisation", with "in vitro" meaning in a lab.

- IUI stands for "intrauterine insemination", a procedure in which sperm is inserted directly into a woman's womb.

- ICSI stands for "intracytoplasmic sperm injection", a procedure in which a single sperm is injected directly into an extracted egg, in a lab.

- According to the HFEA: "Average IVF pregnancy rates using fresh embryo transfers for patients aged 18–34 were 41% per embryo transferred, compared to 6% for patients aged 43–50 when using their own eggs in 2021."

CHAPTER SEVEN

HOW PREGNANCY WORKS

So the fertility treatment works. Or maybe, just straight up, honest-to-goodness *fertility* works?

Anyway.

You're pregnant.

Happily so.

Yay!

What next?

My first close-up experience of pregnancy was when my mum had my youngest sister – 11 years (give or take a fortnight) after she had me. My memory of that pregnancy is profoundly 80s-tinged: pastel legwarmers and hazy excitement, mild-to-moderate concern for my mother's health. (I was a worrier, then.) We had builders in, extending the attic so there'd be enough room for us all. One of them was *absurdly* handsome. "Come On Eileen" knocked "Fame" off the top of the charts, I was sad about that, but the builders were delighted, teased me about it endlessly. My sister was born (born happy actually, happy to her bones, as can be the case with the youngest and unexpected). I was charmed, but also revolted by the stub of severed umbilical cord that clung to her belly button like a gross slug for a week or so after she came home. I can still see it now when I close my eyes.

My second close-up experience of pregnancy was that of my

best friend; one of the first in my university friendship group to have a baby. She broke the news to me and our other best friend when the three of us were on holiday together. We'd just arrived in Paxos; friend two and I were puzzled re why she wasn't immediately drinking.

She told us.

Friend two and I were *appalled*.

"No, you're not," I said, because denial is the first stage of a horrible, graceless response to learning your mate is happily up the duff.

"F*CK OFF!" said friend two, before stropping off for a fag, having gone straight to the *second* stage of a horrible and graceless response to learning your mate is up the duff, i.e. anger.

"I never have to worry you two aren't telling me the truth, do I?" said pregnant friend. Fair to say, this was not her first rodeo on us being a bit odd, rude and generally inappropriate.

We came around to the idea as she got bigger. Ish. "It's kicking!" she told me when we met for lunch. "Dear GOD!" I said. She went into labour the night she and I went to the cinema together. It was snowing. We'd gone to see *Caché* (*très bien!*); she'd shifted about in her seat a bit, but hadn't said anything (she's very stoic). She was in a maternity ward by midnight, and Agnes, my goddaughter, to whom this book is dedicated, and whom (despite an admittedly inauspicious start on a Greek island) I have come to hold in very high regard, popped out a little bit later.

Ah.

Yes, fair point.

I can see that, while this may be a vaguely entertaining insight into my historical – let's call it "hands off" approach to pregnancy

– it can't exactly be considered useful.

Time, I think, to call a midwife.

THE MIDWIFE'S PERSPECTIVE ON PREGNANCY

Well, technically *zoom* a midwife. It is the 2020s, after all.

Anna Kent has practised as a nurse and midwife in the most extraordinary circumstances – and she has experienced maternity services herself, in the most extreme of circumstances. A registered nurse "for over 20 years, now", she did an undergraduate master's degree in nursing in Nottingham and a diploma in Tropical Nursing in London. "I worked in A&E for five years, then went into overseas medical aid, working for Doctors Without Borders. "I did it with the hope of helping people – but it's never that simple." She and I speak – me, from London, she, from her home, in Weymouth, in Dorset – a year after the publication of her first book, *Frontline Midwife* (2022), a raw memoir which delves deep into the never-that-simple business of aid work. While she was based in South Sudan, having trained as a nurse in the UK: "A woman came to us in the full throes of labour and delivered triplets vaginally. And although we did everything we could to help, and she survived, and the triplets survived, an amazing story of survival against all odds, I really recognised that my midwifery skills were not as the woman deserved. Everyone deserves access to a fully qualified midwife. Eight hundred women die in the world, every day, just because of pregnancy, mostly from having no access to a midwife."

Kent returned to the UK, where she qualified as a midwife – "I got a First, which I was really pleased about" – then went on to work in frontline aid missions to Haiti and Bangladesh. Later, in 2015, she briefly taught on "Bangladesh's first ever midwifery course, because before, it wasn't recognised as an autonomous profession in its own right. The course has had really good outcomes, and those midwives are now fully qualified."

Kent also met a bloke in Bangladesh. "My now-ex-husband. He was my surfing instructor. We got pregnant quickly. As with nearly half of births, it was unplanned." A report published in 2022 by UNFPA, the UN's agency for sex and reproductive health, confirms that "Nearly half of all pregnancies, totalling 121 million each year throughout the world, are unintended."[36]

"We had sex once, the condom came off, I was pregnant. We were in love, we got married – but sadly I miscarried that baby. That was a big wake-up call. I'd worked in A&E, where people had presented with miscarriages, I'd worked in maternity services across the world, where a lot of people experienced miscarriages, but I'd really underestimated how brutal a miscarriage can be. Not for everybody. For some people, with their circumstances, it may be a relief. Everybody's experience of pregnancy is their own story to tell. But I found it brutal, because it was a wanted baby. And I'd essentially married a stranger because of this pregnancy." Kent got pregnant again after a month. "That baby – my daughter – died of a brain tumour at six months of pregnancy. Although I'd worked in conflict zones and refugee camps and I'd seen manifestations of how things can go wrong in the most bizarre and extreme ways, my own baby died of something I'd never heard of, a really rare brain tumour called a cerebral

---

36 Nearly half of all pregnancies are unintended – a global crisis, says new UNFPA report, *UNFPA*, 2022 – https://www.unfpa.org/press/nearly-half-all-pregnancies-are-unintended-global-crisis-says-new-unfpa-report

teratoma, literally one in a million. This experience taught me lots of lessons. One was, if I was a pregnant woman in a conflict zone with no access to a midwife, that pregnancy would definitely have killed me." By this point she was back in the UK. "So, though I still grieve the loss of my daughter, I recognise that there were at least 10 ways the NHS saved my life through that pregnancy and birth, including from a haemorrhage after the birth. I am grateful for that care."

Kent would go on to have another daughter – Aisha, six years old by the time Kent and I speak – and to work in the UK, "as a specialist midwife for young parents, complex pregnancies and people who are smoking in pregnancy. I fell into midwifery through aid work highlighting how important it is for everyone to have access to a highly skilled midwife. I ended up absolutely loving it."

Well – I say to Kent – you're definitely as good a person as any in the whole damn world to ask, so: what is a midwife?

"The role of the midwife can be extremely varied and far reaching. A midwife is a medical professional that works with women and birthing people throughout their pregnancy, throughout their birth, throughout the postnatal period, which is the time after giving birth." Typically, this postnatal period of working with a midwife lasts for up to four weeks after birth. "In different cultures and countries the role of the midwife may vary. For a woman in a refugee camp in Bangladesh, her only access to medical care may be a midwife from an aid organisation, so that one midwife has to have an extensive set of skills. Whereas the role of a midwife in most healthcare structures in America may be as an assistant to the doctors, an obstetric nurse rather than a midwife." Midwives practise autonomously, obstetric nurses might not.

The French for "midwife", I learn, is "*sage femme*", which directly translates as "wise woman". The English term originally appears in Middle English, around the 14th century; and the "mid" means "with", as in, it's nothing to do with *being* a wife, everything to do with being *with* the wife, the woman, when she needs support through pregnancy and labour. "You can have male midwives," Kent tells me. "I've worked with some amazing male midwives... Actually, we shouldn't call them 'male midwives', they should just be 'midwives', but for clarity, people often refer to themselves as 'male'."

Right, so: how does it work? Logistically? Practically? Break it down for me: midwifery for the absolute amateur.

"The first time I meet people in pregnancy tends to be when they're about eight weeks pregnant, though the earlier in pregnancy the better. The ideal model of care is continuity of care, the same person, or at least, the same small number of people, will look after a woman or pregnant person throughout their entire pregnancy and birth." Continuity of care, Kent explains, has a positive impact on both the woman and the midwife. First, women tend to like seeing the same people, but it also makes the job more enjoyable for the midwife, which means they're more likely to stay in the profession. This means it benefits from increasingly experienced, increasingly skilled practitioners; it increases women's trust in midwifery generally, on top of which, a midwife is more likely to notice nuanced and really subtle changes in a person, which results in better outcomes for pregnancies. Unfortunately, the Royal College of Midwives' most recent available report into the state of maternity services in

England estimates it's currently around 2500 midwives short. Published in 2023,[37] it also exposes quite breathtaking regional inequalities regarding live births and healthy BMIs of mothers, with much, much better figures recorded for both in London and the southeast. More awful yet, a 2022 report[38] from the RCM notes: "Babies of Black African, Black Caribbean, Pakistani and Bangladeshi ethnicity are much more affected by the higher rates of stillbirth and neonatal death associated with deprivation when compared with their white counterparts."

"To improve things, we need improved training for midwives, and for us to understand any of our own unconscious biases," says Kent.

"For the first time ever," Kent continues, "the RCM reports that we've got fewer midwives coming into the profession than are leaving." This shortfall makes continuity of care infinitely less likely. "But I am really fortunate with my role. I do provide continuity of care to my best ability."

Back to the process. You meet most women at eight weeks?

"The pathway in my area of the UK is: women self-refer into maternity services when they're pregnant. You don't have to go to the GP for a pregnancy test, or any confirmation of pregnancy, to get into the system. The urine pregnancy tests from a GP are as accurate as the £1 pregnancy tests you can buy in cheap shops."

Pregnancy tests work, I'm told, by picking up on a hormone released by the placenta: hCG, human chorionic gonadotropin.

---

37 State of maternity services, Royal College of Midwives, 2023 – https://rcm.org.uk/wp-content/uploads/2024/06/england-soms-2023.pdf

38 Impact of social and ethnic inequalities clear in latest MBRRACE-UK report, Royal College of Midwives, 2022 – rcm.org.uk/media-releases/2022/10/impact-of-social-and-ethnic-inequalities-clear-in-latest-mbrrace-uk-report-says-rcm/

hCG helps thicken the womb lining to support a growing embryo and also instructs the body to stop having periods. hCG levels rise after conception and continue to increase, until about 10 weeks into pregnancy.

"Raised hCG usually indicates a pregnancy – with a little asterisk because there can be rare manifestations such as types of tumour, which show an increase in hCG," Kent says.

Kent explains that the hCG test is a lateral flow test, a strip test, onto which you pee. However, this bit, I already know. I may be child free, but I've done my fair share of panicked pregnancy tests, peed on my fair share of strips. I've got a mate who worked for a while in a big Tesco, his work station was near the women's loos. He would tell me how he watched at least one woman a day walk hastily into those loos, a Tesco bag clutched to her chest, then emerge seven or so minutes later, in tears – of relief, joy or fear. He used to try and guess which one it'd be.

So, women self-refer to maternity services after a pregnancy is confirmed by a home pregnancy test, which they are generally motivated to do because they "may have missed a period," or because "they may also have had some symptoms of pregnancy such as nausea. Some people describe that their nipples feel like they're being brushed with stinging nettles."

Kent tells me this stinging sensation can be similar to the one women experience when their breast milk starts flowing through the milk ducts to the nipples. It's a consequence, she thinks, of a mixture of hormones, specifically oestrogen and prolactin.

And what about morning sickness? Ah, but Kent rails against this kind of nausea being referred to as "morning sickness", because:

While some people may not experience morning sickness at all, others will get it, not just in the morning, and not just for the "morning" of their pregnancy – the earliest stages – but 24 hours a day, sometimes for the entirety of their pregnancy.

Kent feels particularly passionate about this, because that's what happened to her. "I described it as like I had the worst hangover, and none of the fun to warrant it. I would wake up at three in the morning and still be nauseous."

The most extreme form of nausea in pregnancy is hyperemesis gravidarum (HG) a debilitating pregnancy complication which causes extreme nausea and vomiting, and can sometimes be associated with hospitalisation.

Whatever we're calling it, it turns out the reasons for sickness and nausea in pregnancy are not completely understood. Hormonal turbulence is presumed to be at least partly responsible. Kent thinks that because it does most generally affect women in the first 12 weeks of pregnancy, it could also be a protective measure, as the baby is at its most vulnerable stage of development. "So one theory would be that in those early weeks, if you're feeling nauseous, you don't feel like skydiving or motor racing. All you want to do is stay in bed and watch TV and eat bland food."

Should you stay in bed and eat bland food in the early stages of pregnancy?

"We do recognise that good diet in pregnancy is really important. We've got loads of advice about diet in early pregnancy. From my personal experience, I had an app that said: 'Why don't you try hummus and broccoli sticks?' But the thought of anything textured going down my throat – even the thought of it – would make me heave. I was eating floppy white bread with margarine; it certainly helped me appreciate that not all medical advice is necessarily helpful for an individual at that moment."

The RCM has a series of recommendations on nutrition in pregnancy. Before you become pregnant, it advises that you increase your intake of certain micronutrients, specifically folic acid (in supplement form), vitamin D, calcium and iron, all of which are in high demand to support a pregnancy, all of which may be taken in the form of supplements. It continues to advise that both you and your partner eat a balanced and varied diet, that includes plenty of fruit and vegetables, iron-rich protein foods (like lean meat, eggs, lentils) and oily fish (at least one portion a week of salmon, trout, mackerel or sardines); though you should apparently avoid shark, swordfish and marlin, and limit tuna, both fresh and canned, because of its high mercury content. You should eat low-fat dairy products, choose healthier snacks, avoid caffeine and alcohol and stop smoking; and both you and your partner should do all of this because good nutrition will improve the health of his sperm, as well as your body, as you prepare it for a possible pregnancy. Kent's role also involves helping women to stop smoking in pregnancy. "Smoking is the biggest modifiable factor, it directly causes an increased chance of miscarriage, pre-term birth, smaller and sicker babies, still-birth and neonatal deaths."

The Royal College of Midwives continues to recommend that, once pregnant, you take all precautions to limit your chances of developing food poisoning – salmonella, listeria or toxoplasmosis – all of which can have a negative impact on pregnancy, even leading to stillbirth or miscarriage. You do this by cooking all meat and poultry well and completely, drinking only pasteurised or UHT milk and stringently avoiding products made from unpasteurised goat's or sheep's milk, like cheese. The same goes for eggs – although Lion-stamped eggs can be eaten raw or soft-cooked in the UK. Cooked chilled meats should be reheated thoroughly ("ensure they are piping hot") and raw foods should be stored separately from ready-to-eat foods. You should wash your hands thoroughly before and after handling any food, after going to the loo, and before eating, and limit your caffeine intake to 200mg a day.

While we're on the subject of food:

"We know that obesity can have a negative impact on pregnancy – including an increased chance of stillbirth – and we have clinical guidance around this," Kent tells me. "However, it's really important women do not feel judged about their weight, that they feel respected and dignified within maternity services. I work within public health, which covers obesity services. Twenty three per cent of pregnant people nationally are clinically obese, and less than half have a statistically healthy BMI. So we've got almost half with a raised BMI."

Although, she adds, it's not actually that straightforward, because: "There are questions around how accurate a BMI itself is for gauging health. Furthermore, there's no guidance that recommends losing weight in pregnancy, therefore our support is aimed at encouraging healthy activity in pregnancy and offering interventions for the potential risks, such as medications to reduce risks of blood clots." The only real way to tackle obesity in pregnancy is to tackle obesity in the population, so that women are already a healthy weight when they get pregnant.

"One of my friends lost weight in pregnancy," Kent tells me, "just because she used to drink two pints of cider every night, then, during pregnancy, she stopped. Her healthy end of pregnancy weight was less than her starting weight."

That would be one way to do it.

Oh, and on this note, Kent points out that: "No amount of alcohol is safe in pregnancy."

It's also worth mentioning that certain vaccines are recommended during pregnancy – not just to protect you, but to pass early immunity on to your baby. These include the whooping cough vaccine (ideally between 16–32 weeks), the RSV vaccine (offered in the third trimester, between 28–32 weeks), and the flu and COVID-19 vaccines, which are safe at any stage. Most of these use inactivated viruses, so they won't cause infection but help your baby build protection before birth.

As for exercise during pregnancy, Dr Alison Wright, the gynaecologist we met in Chapter 4, tells me thinking has changed considerably on this, relatively recently. Some years ago, she says, "One of my first bosses once said to a woman, who had been experiencing complications: 'For this pregnancy, you're an incubator on legs.' I found that very offensive." The patient had been told to stay in bed, which, unsurprisingly, she was finding difficult. "We would not tell her to stay in bed now."

There is, Dr Wright tells me, no evidence for not exercising while pregnant.

"We generally suggest that people are as active as they want to be, with the proviso they can more easily injure themselves."

Your ligaments become more relaxed in pregnancy. The hormone relaxin makes them more pliable and stretchy, which

means you're more likely to overextend something, destabilise a joint, tear something, dislodge something.

"Do you remember Posh Spice got a lot of flak for wearing high heels when pregnant?" Dr Wright says.

I do. The former Spice Girl, current fashion designer, Victoria Beckham, wore very high heels through the course of all four of her pregnancies, to the consternation of the media. I wrote at least five pieces on it myself. *At least.*

"Actually, there's no harm to the baby in [wearing heels]. But it does mean that, should you fall…"

You'd be at greater risk of injuring yourself?

"Yes." Dr Wright goes on to tell me that a lot of people assume lighter, "gentler" exercising is more appropriate in pregnancy – some yoga, nice gentle stretching – but that this isn't necessarily at all true. Exercises like yoga can potentially stretch round the core and the pelvic ligaments; certain poses can put a lot of pressure on your belly, or engage your abdominals too forcefully. It is crucial to make sure your yoga class is appropriate for pregnancy, not just assume yoga is by definition gentle.

"For pregnancy, one of the challenges, which makes it interesting, but also frustrating," says Dr Wright, "is that we don't have data and research. It's not ethical to say: 'You – run a marathon every day while you're pregnant. You – lie down and watch TV. We'll see how healthy your respective babies are…' It's very difficult ethically to put pregnant women into randomised controlled trials."

Mainly, Dr Wright believes the emphasis still needs to be on changing how we think about the bodies of pregnant women. "Historically, women have been told they're just vehicles for the baby," and that's the reason why they have to be mindful of ourselves physically, when in fact they need to be careful of their own bodies because *"they're their own bodies!"*.

Next, I learn that a developing pregnancy has four early, progressive stages, the **zygote**, the fertilised cell, the ground zero of a pregnancy; the **blastocyst**, the cluster of dividing cells, which forms five to six days after that egg is fertilised by a sperm; the **embryo**, which is when the blastocyst is enfolded in an amniotic sac at around day 10 to 12; and the foetus, to which the embryo graduates in its ninth week (or the 11th week after your last period). These first 12 weeks are also referred to as the **first trimester** of pregnancy.

The **second trimester** is weeks 13–27, when you become visibly pregnant; the **third** and final **trimester** covers weeks 28–40.

"Did you know you don't have to legally seek any medical advice in pregnancy?" Anna Kent asks me. "Until the baby is born, it doesn't have legal rights."

I did not know that. Why might people not seek medical care?

"Different reasons. Sometimes, people don't trust the NHS and sometimes people don't trust Western medicine, sometimes people don't require it. They may not want scans or blood tests. And actually, we have to remember that that woman? She's got legal rights, legal autonomy over her body. If it's an informed choice and people are opting out, it's their legal right." However, she goes on, it might also be that there are other issues at play. Safeguarding concerns, issues around alcohol, drugs, domestic abuse. "If someone isn't accessing medical care, it would be very sensible for us to explore why."

This, Kent tells me, is called "professional curiosity, where we do ask the complicated questions." The approach, then, is to balance the asking of such questions, with the developing of a good rapport, while effectively communicating that she, Kent, will not do anything at all to someone's body without first receiving their informed consent.

Informed consent is defined as "permission granted in full knowledge of the possible consequences, typically that which is given by a patient to a doctor for treatment with knowledge of the possible risks and benefits." Kent explains that this is the case, "even if I'm taking blood pressure, or a urine sample, all the things the medical services may think is just routine care, I gain consent to do so."

She tells me that the taking of blood pressure during pregnancy is essential, because pregnancy itself can cause pre-eclampsia, high blood pressure, and that can be fatal if it's undetected, and progresses to eclampsia – a medical emergency. It is, I learn, quite common; in the UK, around one to five pregnant women out of every 100 can develop pre-eclampsia, though mildly. Around one in 200 is at risk of developing it severely.

Pre-eclampsia doesn't tend to manifest before 24 weeks, but Kent will measure blood pressure at the routine eight- to twelve-week check; because women may be living with high blood pressure before becoming pregnant without realising it. If you have high blood pressure, diabetes or kidney disease when you become pregnant, you're at a greater risk of developing pre-eclampsia later in that pregnancy.

At the eight-week booking appointment, Kent also tests a client's urine. She's looking, she says, for signs of infection, as well as further clues on blood pressure. High protein in urine, for example, can indicate a rise in blood pressure because pre-eclampsia can damage blood vessels in the kidneys, which means they can leak protein into the urine – protein which usually stays in the blood.

She also checks the woman's heart rate, and for a regular heart rhythm. Cardiac disease, I learn, is the highest direct cause of maternal deaths in the UK. Women do still die in childbirth here. According to most recently available figures published in the BMJ, the *British Medical Journal*: "In 2020–22 there were 13.41 deaths in every 100,000 maternities." Furthermore, according to a report from MBRRACE-UK, published in 2023:[39] "There remains a two-fold difference in maternal mortality rates for Black women compared to White women. Asian women also had a slightly increased risk compared to White women. Women living in the most deprived areas continued to have a maternal mortality rate twice that of women living in the least deprived areas."

Which is devastating.

"Nationally, we do have some deaths," confirms Kent. "Every one of those is an absolute tragedy that needs understanding; they're all thoroughly investigated and the findings disseminated nationally. We're still one of the safest places globally to be pregnant and give birth – but currently we recognise the significant challenges faced by many maternity services and it is our responsibility to keep fighting to create a safe place for women

---

39 Maternal mortality 2021-2023, MBRRACE-UK, 2023 – https://www.npeu. ox.ac.uk/mbrrace-uk/data-brief/maternal-mortality-2021-2023

and birthing people. Out of all the women that died in the UK, the highest direct cause of death was cardiac disease, stroke, blood clots and suicide."

Kent confirms the fact that Shazia Malik told me, about the importance of screening for STIs. She offers all women screening for HIV, Hepatitis B and syphilis. All of these tests are done through blood samples, and all are optional. "You don't legally have to do any of this," she says, although she really hopes you will. She goes on to tell me that if you know a pregnant woman is HIV positive, you have a really good chance of ensuring the virus isn't passed on to the baby. Kent knows this first hand, because she spent some time in the UK as an HIV specialist midwife.

Gosh, that really is incredible, I say, and so hopeful. How is that achieved? "Most of the time, through anti-retroviral drugs. Which is really exciting. There is still a small amount of transmission. When I was working in Nottingham, one lady presented late in pregnancy, so she had a high viral load, and the baby was already infected. Babies can become infected through breast milk as well." But you can, she says, almost fully eradicate mother-to-baby transmission of HIV if you know about it early enough. Screening for chlamydia and gonorrhoea – recommended for all pregnant women under 25, and done with a self-testing vaginal swab – will also help protect the baby from becoming infected in labour. These infections live in the vagina, so there's a chance the baby will pick them up on its way out, during a vaginal birth.

"Congenital chlamydia and gonorrhoea can cause lung and eye infections for the baby, which when I worked in conflict areas could be so bad they could cause blindness," and also, potentially, "sterility [in the mother], miscarriage and pre-term birth."

Another thing Anna Kent is checking for, another thing about which she must show "professional curiosity", is the possibility of domestic abuse. "Because we know one in four women experiences it in their lifetime, and for a third of them, we think, it starts in pregnancy."

So we are particularly vulnerable to domestic abuse when pregnant?

"Yes. What I tend to do is start by explaining what domestic abuse is and how it can manifest, as not everyone is aware that they themselves are in an abusive relationship. There are four main types of abuse: physical, sexual, emotional (including coercive control) and financial. Then I'll ask them sensitively: 'Do you feel like any of those are affecting you? Do you feel safe at home? Is there anyone you know who could be a risk to you or your baby?' We know that often people need repeated conversations before they may disclose abuse, so I'm aiming to create an environment where, if anything were to change, they understand I would be a safe place to go to. I will ask these questions again throughout pregnancy and postnatally, as often as it is safe to do so."

Historically, she tells me, people have been nervous about telling midwives about problems in their lives around alcohol, drugs or domestic abuse, because ultimately they're concerned about their child being removed from their care. "My role is to encourage working with other services like social care or addiction services if they are recommended, as it demonstrates a desire to improve things."

Midwives also ask questions concerning other, sensitive issues, mental health and female genital mutilation (FGM), among them. FGM is a procedure which involves partial or total removal of the external female genitalia, or injury to genitalia for non-medical purposes. Kent has worked with women who experienced FGM most commonly in her aid work, but points out that, because "we do see women with FGM in the UK," and because there are risks posed to a woman and her baby in pregnancy from FGM, it is important to have a non-judgemental conversation with all "people who are pregnant," so that "they have the highest level of maternity care."

Equally: "If people decide they don't want to continue with the pregnancy, they want to have a termination, then my role is, not to counsel them specifically, but to refer them to supportive services and offer them a safe place to be able to explore their feelings, a non-judgemental place." Abortion is legal in the UK up until 24 weeks of pregnancy; the vast majority – 89% according to most recent figures – happen before 10 weeks.

How many times Kent sees a woman during a pregnancy depends on a number of factors. NICE, the National Institute for Health and Care Excellence, recommends that midwives see people "about 11 times during pregnancy", though Kent tends to see her clients more because they often have complex needs.

The first time she sees them is at "booking", which tends to happen at eight weeks, though can be later. Next, they're offered a 12-week scan, which is when she assesses whether there is a heartbeat and finds out where the pregnancy is implanted, and if that place is safe: "because you can get pregnant outside the uterus. Ectopic pregnancies."

According to the website of the Royal College of Obstetricians and Gynaecologists, one in 90 UK pregnancies is ectopic; most develop in the fallopian tubes, but in rare cases, they can develop elsewhere. Diagnosis is made through an assessment of symptoms, through examination, blood tests and scans. Treatments vary, though, sadly, to the same end: termination. An ectopic pregnancy is simply never viable; the foetus or developing embryo cannot possibly survive and needs to be removed before it causes harm to the woman carrying it. If left, it can cause internal bleeding and death. It's the most common cause of maternal mortality in the first trimester.

The 12-week scan is often the point at which women discover how many babies they're expecting, just the one, or twins, triplets or more. Women will also be offered screening for Edwards' syndrome, Patau's syndrome and Down's syndrome. During this assessment, medical professionals can establish the percentage chance of a baby having chromosomal abnormalities, through a combination of blood tests and observations of the scan, such as the thickness at the back of the baby's neck. An increased measurement may indicate a higher risk of certain conditions like Down's Syndrome.

Scans in pregnancy also look for other differences, for example, spina bifida, which, according to the NHS site, "is when a baby's spine and spinal cord do not develop properly in the womb, causing a gap in the spine." Taking folic acid supplements – as the RCM, the NHS and pretty much every medical body you care to consult recommend – is crucial in helping prevent spina bifida, especially before pregnancy and during its early stages, because it helps the neural tube, which becomes the brain and spine, to develop.

Kent will next see her pregnant clients at 16 weeks for routine checks, more urine, more blood pressure. "I sit and go through the results of the 12-week scan, because not everyone understands it straight away. I review with them their individualised care plan and discuss further if I recommend for them to see a consultant in pregnancy or further screening tests for things like gestational diabetes – diabetes caused by pregnancy."

Most pregnant women are next seen by a midwife at about 25 weeks, though Kent tells me she tends to see people at 20 weeks, because of the particular nature of her work.

After 20 weeks, midwives can listen in to the foetal heart rate with a Pinard stethoscope (which looks like a listening horn) and a handheld doppler (an electronic device that uses soundwaves). "It is not recommended for women to buy their own doppler online and listen at home, as there have been very sad cases where babies have died because women have misinterpreted what they have heard, and not sought medical help when they needed it."

At each appointment, midwives continue to look for some of the signs and symptoms of potential problems, such as pre-eclampsia, or obstetric cholestasis, a liver issue, which can cause it to produce excess bile acids, and increase the risk of stillbirth. "The symptoms of it are strange," Kent says. "People often get a really odd itching on the palms of their hands and the soles of their feet. So we discuss these symptoms, because, on a hot day, could this be obstetric cholestasis? Could this be because I'm hot and sweaty? Have I changed my detergent? So our advice is to call for advice if you are worried about this (and other) symptoms."

In pregnancy, Kent tells me, people have access to a 24/7 maternity advice line – though the name and number for this varies depending on your hospital and trust.

"Women and pregnant people are offered a scan at around 20 weeks of pregnancy," Kent tells me, the point at which you can opt to find out about the gender of your unborn child (although, she points out, not all units offer that service). She tells me there can be a differing of understanding of this scan between medical professionals and expectant families, because, while they're often excited to know the gender, effectively celebrating the pregnancy, medical staff are scanning for anomalies. "It's called 'the anomaly scan'. What we're doing is looking in depth, all the way through, the baby…"

Kent slices through the air in front of her with her hands, at minuscule intervals, up and down the length of an imaginary foetus.

"Looking at their organs, looking at their brain, looking at the length of their legs. Looking at their bones, the width of their belly. Literally going, bit by bit, really carefully, through the baby. We're looking for any potential *problems*."

It is, she says, really important that people understand that. Again, it's part of "informed consent". If they don't want to know the results of such examinations, it's important they consider that before the scan is done.

It was at the 20-week scan that Kent found out about her first daughter's brain tumour, when she understood her second pregnancy couldn't continue without putting her own life at risk.

"I can still remember the language used. I'm not very good at reading scans, even though I've been a midwife for 12 years – I'm not a sonographer. It did feel like she was taking a long time with the head. But I was just really excited, because I could see my baby's little toes wriggling, her little hands moving... And then the sonographer went back to scan the head again, and I was lying there thinking: 'Maybe this is normal? I don't really know.' All she said was this: 'I don't know how to tell you this, Anna...' And suddenly, my world imploded and would forever be different. Even though, as a trained professional, I knew the point of that scan was to look for anomalies – I was there as a mum, excited about seeing my baby's toes wriggling."

As desperate as this is, as unimaginably painful, it has also made Kent think a great deal about something which she tells me midwives, obstetricians and gynaecologists weigh up constantly: how far do we go in explaining the risks of pregnancy to someone who is pregnant, versus the need not to freak them the hell out, or harm them. This, Kent tells me, involves discussion about individual wishes. "It depends how they feel about risks. Some people prefer to know about all risks and set their mind up that it could happen, some people prefer not to hear anything at all."

Discussing risk, she says, is always an unbelievably fine balance. Some midwives, she says, prefer to use the word "chance" rather than "risk" – the word itself can have negative connotations. "Some people accuse midwives of infantilising them by not telling them everything, *every* risk. Like: one in eight pregnancies for, I think it's under 30-year-olds, ends in miscarriage, however, even the data varies."

(According to the NHS website, "Miscarriages are much more common than most people realise. It's thought around one in eight known pregnancies will end in miscarriage. Many miscar-

234

riages happen before someone knows they're pregnant."[40])

"So when someone comes to me for a booking," Kent goes on, "am I being fair if I say: 'Congratulations! You're pregnant! How brilliant. There is a one in eight possibility your pregnancy could miscarry...' Whilst this is an accurate explanation of risk – that is not how most people would choose to start their working relationship with their midwife. But then, if she does go on to miscarry, and I haven't had this conversation, then there's more harm potentially from that miscarriage... This conversation is constantly evolving."

As a pregnancy continues, as it goes on into its third trimester, when classically, tiredness and discomfort feature more and more, along with heartburn and indigestion, back pain from hefting the rapidly increasing bump around, puffiness in the face, wrists, and ankles... Kent introduces conversations about the practicalities of giving birth, and information around breastfeeding.

Ideally, she tells me, women go to antenatal classes. This, according to the available data, has really positive outcomes in terms of how prepared and informed women feel. Kent points out, however, that not everyone, in every part of the country, has access to antenatal classes – and even if they do, not all people like or trust group settings.

In her clinic, she has props: a doll, a pelvis, a cervix, even a knitted boob. You've got to meet people where they're at, she explains. "Some people have never ever heard of a placenta before. Some people have done loads of research and know

---

40 Miscarriage overview, NHS, 2025 – https://www.nhs.uk/conditions/miscarriage/

extensive information. It's about communicating effectively to your audience in a way that's helpful to them. Many of the people I work with may not have English as a first language, or may have additional learning needs. I have to take all that into account with our conversations."

With regard to her overseas aid work, while the fact most people birthed at home due to lack of access to healthcare was, in many respects, far less than ideal, it did mean that their female relatives, their sisters and their daughters, were extremely well versed in labour, because they would see it first hand, often many times over, before they themselves became pregnant. "They witnessed birth," Kent says, "and sometimes death, which, though always awful, did also mean, when they themselves were pregnant, that they were very aware of the risks – they'd seen them, they'd smelled them, they'd witnessed it."

In the UK, relatively, of course, we're sometimes ignorant of how pregnancy and labour unfurl, until it's happening to us. Help, advice and awareness come in unexpected forms, however.

"We do have [Channel 4 documentary series] *One Born Every Minute*, and we do have [BBC drama] *Call the Midwife* – and that has helped some of the national dialogue. We rarely used to talk about pre-eclampsia, but then an episode of *Call the Midwife* did, and the term is now more widely known; people do want to talk about it. They ask me about things they've seen on the last episode. And the positives of *One Born Every Minute* – although it doesn't always show midwives in a realistic light, they have far more time than we do to have tea and cake – it shows people puffing, panting and being really vocal. Labour can be beautiful and sparkly lights and rose petals and calm, but that's not all labours."

"Some labour is messy, there may be poo and it's bloody and there's birth products. Opening people's minds to what labour can look like – that it's *still* a healthy, positive birth experience can be really important..."

Kent makes it clear everything we've talked about amounts to a brief overview of the care midwives offer to women through their pregnancy, a consideration of some of the themes, but that it is complex and nuanced, so there are aspects to it we haven't contemplated. She does, however, raise the topic of pooing in labour; which is, she says, one of the things women worry about most in pregnancy, so we will revisit it in depth in the following chapter: childbirth.

But first:

THE NEUROSCIENTIST'S PERSPECTIVE

Because apparently, a pregnant brain is a busy one.

Having developed substantially through puberty, through adolescence and into your early 20s, "your brain matter," Dr McKay tells me, from Sydney, "will stay where it is. The next time we see a really dramatic change in women, is pregnancy."

And what does that look like?

"It's another [stage where we see] significant grey matter volume reduction in brain areas involved in social cognition, in reading social cues."

Anyone paying attention will remember that, when Dr McKay and I originally discussed reduction in the brain's grey matter, which first occurs during puberty, she explained it's the process by which the brain gets smarter, sharper. That thinning of grey matter allows for speedier connections between axons, which, in the case of the brain, link neurons.

If, in puberty that thinning of grey matter leads to a "mastery of skills" – particularly in areas like planning and judgement, reasoning, problem solving and critical thinking – in pregnancy, grey matter thins to allow heightened, improved social cognition, specifically designed to improve reading the social cues of a baby.

"Pregnancy is preparing your brain and mind for motherhood. And what do we need to do when a new baby is in our arms, especially if it's a first baby? We need to be able to very quickly learn how to interpret what the baby needs and wants. Initially, it can't tell us. They can cry, and we respond. Or they're really cute. We're drawn to them when they're crying, but we're also drawn to them just because they smell amazing, they've got olfactory cuteness, cheeks that we want to squeeze."

So, our brain changes in pregnancy, to make us more sensitive to, and inclined to respond, to cuteness?

"Yes!"

("From an evolutionary standpoint, cuteness is a very potent protective mechanism that ensures survival for otherwise completely dependent infants," reads a 2016 article, published in *Science Daily*.[41])

This change, Dr McKay says, is driven "particularly in the third trimester" by oestradiol, that especially potent hormonal subtype of oestrogen, which "is at sky-high levels during

---

41   Babies don't just look cute, scientists find, *Trends in Cognitive Sciences*, 2016
– https://www.sciencedaily.com/releases/2016/06/160606115909.htm

pregnancy. If you have a pregnancy, you'll get a thousand times more oestrogen than you'll receive in the entire rest of your life. And that's a good thing, because oestrogen is a good hormone, our brains *really* like it. It builds [brain] resilience, and – particularly during pregnancy – it's driving the social brain rewiring." As in puberty, the brain in pregnancy goes into "a state of plasticity." Meaning? "That it's super sensitive to learning and change." This affects the social brain, particularly the areas involved in empathy, which means that, even if you don't automatically know what to do when your baby is born, your learning curve is much less steep than if you're not a pregnant mother.

Dr McKay knows this because her 2023 book, *Baby Brain,* was based on "a [2017] study, which came from a Spanish lab. Make sure you reference the authors – Elseline Hoekzema, Susanna Carmona and Erika Barba-Müller – they were responsible for the brain-imaging studies of women during their first pregnancy. They scanned women's brains before and immediately after their first pregnancy, and they also scanned men – these were heterosexual couples – so they scanned the fathers' brains, as well, just to see if the changes they saw were due to pregnancy or parenting." And? "They were due to pregnancy."

But this "heightened plasticity and sensitivity to learn and understand your baby's cue" is only "one part of the change." What other changes are there, in the brains of pregnant women?

"There are some that have been picked up in animals, not 100% confirmed in humans," says Dr McKay, though she strongly suspects the same will hold true for us too. "Oxytocin – a hormone released at childbirth, and if you're breastfeeding – probably alters your auditory cortex, the part of your brain that hears sounds." Meaning:

"You're very sensitive to the sound of a baby's cry. So, if you have a baby, and you're sound asleep at night, often you'll suddenly be wide awake, and you'll think: 'Why am I awake?' And then two seconds later, your baby goes: 'MEH!' Every mother will swear they woke up before the baby started crying. What probably happened was, before the baby woke, it started going: 'Mmmm...' And you'll have heard that and it's woken you up. Your husband or your partner will be next to you, snoring away. We know that happens in other mammals."

These changes, this rewiring, Dr McKay thinks, is routinely misconstrued. Pregnant women, and women who have given birth and are now raising newborns, are often assumed to be cognitively lesser, when in fact, they're demonstrably sharper. This, then, is the real definition of "baby brain".

"If we look at how the different parts of the brain connect with each other, and communicate with each other, the brains of mothers are more flexible and efficient and streamlined. It's almost as if they've become changed so that their entire focus, all the attention, your whole being is tuned into this little human that you have to keep alive. Especially for your first baby, you're hypervigilant, you're consumed, your attention is consumed by this little baby. There's a biological mandate for that. Mother nature wants us to keep the baby alive. You're not meant to be thinking about your emails, or what you're having for dinner. You're just meant to keep this little human alive, and so your brain is primed to tune into them."

This effect is lessened, she says, through later pregnancies. "The second baby is very different. You've kind of figured it out. It's like you don't have to go through puberty twice. You are a mother, so you kind of know what to do. Most mothers will say for the second, they're much more relaxed, they're not as on edge. Because you've already figured out what matters. The first baby is when we see the significant neurological change. It's the thinning of those parts of the brain that are involved with reading baby cues, so that's really very meaningful. It's the biggest neurological change we see in adulthood."

All these changes! All these hundreds (thousands?) of precisely and minutely calibrated adaptations and evolutions, these automated precautions and allowances, across every part of us, all so we can perpetuate the species! If it were a machine, it'd blow your freakin' *mind*. But it's a body, it's *our body*! It deserves a design award, don't you think? The Nobel Prize for being just incredibly fit for purpose. Which it wins, over and over and over again. Like Ant and Dec at the National Television Awards.

I know it's been said before, repeated to the point of cliché. Yet it bears repeating: the female body is a *miracle*.

WHAT I KNOW NOW

- Nearly half of all pregnancies worldwide are unplanned.

- The word midwife means "with wife". Midwives are not necessarily women.

- Most commonly, a midwife will meet a pregnant woman at around eight weeks into her pregnancy.

- Continuity of care – where the same midwife, or small group of midwives, attends to the same pregnancy – is the best model for ensuring a good outcome for that pregnancy.

- The regional inequalities of good maternal outcomes in the UK are dramatic and weighted towards the southeast and London. Babies of Black African, Black Caribbean, Pakistani and Bangladeshi ethnicity are much more affected by the higher rates of stillbirth than their white counterparts.

- In the UK, there remains a two-fold difference in maternal mortality rates for Black women compared to White women. Asian women also have a slightly increased risk compared to White women. Women living in the most deprived areas continue to have a maternal mortality rate twice that of women living in the least deprived areas.

- Women are under no legal obligation to seek medical care, advice or support when pregnant. However, most do, self-referring following a positive pregnancy test, or experiencing physical symptoms of pregnancy.

- Pregnancy tests work by picking up elevated levels of the hormone hCG. This is the hormone that helps to thicken the lining of the womb. It also stops periods.

- It's not clear what causes sickness in pregnancy. Best guesses involve some combination of hormonal disruption and a protective function – a woman who is feeling very sick is unlikely to indulge in vigorous activities, which might harm a developing embryo.

- Good nutrition and a well-balanced diet are crucial in pregnancy. Folic acid supplements help reduce the risk of spina bifida. Care should be taken to avoid food poisoning, which can be very harmful to a pregnancy.

- Obesity in pregnancy contributes to maternal death rates. Pregnant women should not attempt to lose weight, but anyone trying to get pregnant will improve their chances dramatically by achieving a healthy weight beforehand.

- Exercising in the same way that you did before you were pregnant, while pregnant, is recommended – with the understanding that some forms of exercise, certain yoga poses, for example, can be harmful to a foetus.

- Pregnancy also tends to make ligaments more pliable, which means they can overstretch and tear, or destabilise a joint.

- Modern medicine means there's now an incredibly high success rate for prevention of mother-to-child transmission of HIV in pregnancy. The earlier medics know about an HIV-positive status, the better the chances of stopping the infection.

- Our brains change when we're pregnant. They become sharper and more acute; every change is designed to make us more attuned to the needs of our baby.

- During pregnancy, a woman's body will be bombarded by a thousand times more oestrogen than it'll receive in the entire rest of her life.

- There's growing evidence that oxytocin, released into women's bodies during labour and when they're breastfeeding, also alters their auditory complex, the part of the brain that hears sound. This may make them incredibly sensitive to their babies' cries and explain why they often report waking up in the night *before* their baby starts crying.

irregular contractions in Later Labour, these may vary in which

CHAPTER EIGHT

HOW CHILDBIRTH WORKS

(According to the women who've done it.
A chapter also known as: "MY F*CKING FANNY!")

I haven't been through childbirth. I've followed the process from afar, and the comfort of my own bed, updated through dramatic nights by frenzied texts from partners and birth partners. I've had a little cry over the: "She's here!", "He's here!" messages. I've produced desperately inappropriate gifts and offers to be there for the first tattoo, just in case anyone thought I was going soft.

But I have never done it myself.

I decide, therefore, to get the NHS's perspective on the process – the official blow-by-blow account of how it happens, how babies enter the world – along with the perspective of a load of my friends.'

You know.

For balance.

According to the NHS website, there are four stages of labour. Before those four, though, comes:

THE LATENT STAGE

During which your cervix begins to soften and dilate, with the end goal of allowing your baby's head to squeeze its way out of your uterus (followed by *the rest of it*). You may, the site says, feel irregular contractions in Latent Labour; these may vary in intensity, from uncomfortable to more painful. Latent Labour can last for hours, possibly even days, before Stage 1, Established Labour, begins.

In Latent Labour, the NHS recommends you have something to eat and drink, that if it starts at night, you try to stay comfortable and relaxed – even sleep (if such a thing is conceivable). If Latent Labour starts during the day, the NHS suggests you stay upright and gently active, which will help "your baby move down into your pelvis" and also help "your cervix to dilate". It recommends breathing exercises, massage, warm baths or showers to help ease pain (TBF I recommend these on any old Tuesday to help ease the pain, pregnant or otherwise).

Next, comes:

STAGE 1: ESTABLISHED LABOUR

This is defined by the NHS as "where your cervix has dilated to about 4cm, and your contractions are stronger and more regular." You'll know you're there, the NHS says, and so should contact your midwife or maternity unit if:

your contractions are kicking in every five minutes or more
OR
your waters break, which means, the embryonic sac which protects the baby while it grows inside the uterus has burst, in preparation for the birth
OR
your contractions are very strong and you think you need pain relief
OR
you're worried about anything.

If you go to hospital before Established Labour has kicked in, and if your pregnancy is otherwise straightforward, there's a chance you'll get packed off back home at least for a bit. But once labour is definitely, 100% established and *on*, you'll be admitted if you're giving birth in hospital.

This is how my friend C experienced Established Labour.

"My waters broke, 5am. I was very lucky, had both my babies at the Portland. Went in, chose my room – 101, same as Diana… Oh no, hang on, [my husband] Mark says it was Fergie! – had breakfast. They told me, I was 4cm dilated…" i.e., C's cervix had opened by 4cm.

10cm is – according to the NHS website – considered to be full dilation, enough for the baby's head to pass from the uterus into the vagina. This process – towards full dilation – takes an average of 8–18 hours on a first labour, but can speed up on subsequent births.

Your midwife (NHS guidance continues) will check on you at regular intervals, see how you're going, offer you support, advice and pain relief should you need it. They'll give you regular vaginal exams to establish how your labour is progressing, how far your cervix is dilating. You do not have to have these exams if you do not want them; you can talk to your midwife about what they are, why they matter, and so forth.

"First baby," says my friend R, "the pain wasn't bad at the start – at least compared to migraines." R suffers with migraines. "But when the pain kicked in, I was given an epidural, which brought the whole process to a close. My cervix stopped dilating."

Epidurals are powerful pain-relieving injections, which go directly into the spine, generally in the first or second stages of labour. They're not appropriate close to delivery.

(They sound incredibly painful, I say, to obstetrician and gynaecologist Dr Alison Wright. "It's uncomfortable having it inserted. But the anaesthetist will give a local anaesthetic first. It has to get into the nerve space around the spinal cord. The epidural space is the space around the nerves which cause pain – or not – to the rest of your body, from the waist down.")

"Epidurals can prolong the second stage of labour," says the NHS. (Although Dr Wright tells me that this occurs far less now with the modern 'mobile' epidurals.)

"I had sudden pre-eclampsia when I went into labour with my first," says T, of the birth of her eldest son. Pre-eclampsia is that potentially highly dangerous increase in blood pressure, which is associated with pregnancy and labour. Was she frightened? "I didn't really know what was going on. My husband was TER-RIFIED. They told him to call my parents, said he may have to choose between baby and mother."

F*CKING HELL.

"Nah, it's fine."

"I was leaking green everywhere when I was admitted," says my friend P. Her waters had broken, just as they should – however, the greenish staining she noticed in them was meconium, evidence her baby had done a poo, something that should only happen after birth, because an unborn baby can breathe it in, which can lead to serious problems.

You and your baby will be monitored throughout labour, the NHS goes on. Medics will apply a small, handheld device to your stomach to listen to your baby's heartbeat every 15 minutes or so; though if you have an epidural, or if there are any concerns about you or your baby, your midwife might suggest they monitor you both through electronic methods. This means strapping two pads to your bump, one of which tracks your contractions continuously; the other, your baby's heartbeat. Sometimes, something poetically called a "foetal scalp electrode" may be attached directly to the baby's head for more accurate monitoring of their heartbeat. It goes in up your vaginal canal, through the cervix, and onto the baby's head. The foetal scalp electrode will only be removed just before the baby is born, unlike the bump pads, which – if they show normal, non-concerning activity – can be removed at any time. Electronic monitoring can restrict how much you move around in labour, which can affect how comfortable you are.

It might well be (the NHS website continues) that your labour is slower than expected, so needs to be sped up. Perhaps your contractions aren't frequent enough or strong enough; perhaps your baby is in an awkward position (please note, this is NHS terminology, not mine. I think, if it *were* me, I'd perhaps point out, none of this is your fault, nor can you be expected to remedy it yourself necessarily, but don't worry: someone medically qualified *will*... But what do I know? I'm neither a medic, nor a mother, and hell: maybe it isn't as inherently judgy as I seem to think).

Onwards.

Labour can, the NHS informs me, be sped up in two ways: either by breaking your waters (assuming they haven't already broken), or with an oxytocin drip. Breaking your waters, also known as ARM, artificial rupture of the membrane, that uterine sac that keeps your baby safe through pregnancy, can, in itself, make your contractions stronger, more vigorous, and regular, which will accelerate labour. It's achieved by making a small break in the membrane during a vaginal exam; if, as intended, this does make your contractions stronger, it may also make them more painful, so your midwife or doctor should talk to you about pain relief in advance.

The oxytocin drip works because your contractions – indeed, the whole of your labour – is activated and controlled by your own oxytocin, your own personal supply of the cuddly love hormone.

In terms of geeing up labour, adding more oxytocin into the mix might provide the boost your contractions need. It goes in through a drip inserted into a vein in your arm or wrist. You'll then be electronically monitored to check your baby is coping with the intensified contractions; plus, vaginal exams, to make sure the drip is helping you dilate.

Once your cervix is dilated by 10cm, you're considered fully dilated, you're reaching the end of the first stage of labour, at which point, you may feel an urge to push.

Welcome to the second stage of labour.

STAGE 2: DELIVERY OF THE BABY

First (says the NHS) your midwife will help you to find a comfortable position from which to give birth. "You may want to sit, lie on your side, stand, kneel, or squat, although…" it adds, with – perhaps this is just me, but I definitely detected a wry tone: "squatting may be difficult if you're not used to it." It suggests you go onto all fours if you've suffered from backache through pregnancy, and also recommends practising some of these positions before labour starts, which seems sensible.

With a fully dilated cervix comes the time to push. This happens because your baby has moved further down the birth canal, towards the entrance to your vagina. The sensation this creates may feel a bit like you need to poo.

You can push during contractions whenever you feel the urge, the NHS continues. You may not feel the urge to push immediately. If you have had an epidural, you may not feel an urge to push at all.

"When it came to pushing," says C, "I was so scared of pooing."

"*So many women are,*" midwife Anna Kent says. Does it happen a lot? In her experience, "it's about 30% of the time. And I would say, if I'm with someone who's giving birth and they poo, I'm thinking: that's often a really positive sign; the birth is likely progressing and the baby's head is pushing onto her rectum."

On top of the fear of pooing, C continues: "I'd had an epidural, so I didn't feel a thing. Every time the doc said 'push!'... Nothing! Some of the time, I pretended to push. Eventually, my baby's heart rate fell, so: ventouse..."

A ventouse is a vacuum cup device that looks a bit like a plunger. It is attached to the baby's head to help pull it out in what the Royal College of Obstetricians refers to as "an assisted vaginal birth". An assisted vaginal birth might also be achieved with forceps. One in eight women in the UK has one, one in three with their first baby.

"And out my daughter popped," says C, "with a big pointy cone head." This is a consequence of vacuum extraction, officially called "caput succedaneum" or "scalp oedema". It usually settles down within days. I have one mate who called her newborn daughter "Cone Head the Baby-barian" on account of it.

This stage of labour, the NHS points out (again, I suspect, a touch wryly? Can an NHS website *be* wry? TBD), is hard work. ("It was also a bloodbath," says another friend. "Bet the NHS doesn't mention *that* on the website, does it?" I concede, it does not.)

It should take around three hours for a first baby, the NHS thinks, up to two, for subsequent babies.

"I had my third child in the US, that's where we were living at the time," says K. "Even though it was my third, I remember pushing and pushing and saying 'I can't do this. I can't…' I remember looking at my big bump belly, which hadn't moved, and actually thinking: 'What if I'm the first woman on earth who can't get her baby out, and I have to leave the hospital still pregnant? What happens then? Do I come back? How long can a not-birthed baby stay alive in the womb?'" Her son was eventually born with a ventouse. "Another cone head!"

Next up: your baby is born. This is *still*, apparently, merely the second stage of labour. When your baby's head is about to emerge, says the NHS, your midwife will ask you to stop pushing, and instead, take some short breaths, which you expel out through your mouth. "This is so your baby's head can be born slowly and gently, giving the skin and muscles in the area between your vagina and anus (the perineum) time to stretch."

It may not stretch enough, however, which might warrant an episiotomy, a medical cut in the flesh between the vagina and the bum, administered to prevent that flesh tearing. "We *really* want to avoid tearing," obstetrician/gynaecologist Dr Alison Wright tells me. "Potentially, those tears can go all the way down to the anus, a third- or fourth-degree tear – that's what we need to avoid."

Dr Wright says you can help minimise your risk of tearing by massaging your perineum before labour, during pregnancy.

Literally, just massage it?

"Yup. You can get devices, there's something called 'Epi-No' on the internet, which can stretch [the flesh] mechanically, but it works just as well with massage. Use oil. Anything. In some cultures, they [massage] during the birth, which I've started to encourage people to do, I think it works well to try and prevent getting tears." Crucially, Dr Wright says, we should: "Talk to women [before labour] about the possibility of perineal tears. It's a real bugbear of mine. Some people don't like to talk to women antenatally about anything that might go wrong, because it could scare them – but I think that's really paternalistic. And it's not ethical, because there's something they can do about it. You need to say [in advance of labour]: 'That's the anus, that's the vagina, those are the labia, this is the perineum here, and what we really want to avoid is a tear that goes from there to there… So we do a small cut to the side.' Then it doesn't comes as a complete shock to someone: 'I'm just about to do a cut here, is that OK with you?'"

The NHS site says: "You'll be given a local anaesthetic injection to numb the area before the cut is made. Once your baby is born, an episiotomy, or any large tears, will be stitched closed." It is crucial to care for that wound after the birth, given its proximity to germ-propagating issues like your bum. You can use an ice pack to reduce the swelling, and squirt it with warm water through a "peri bottle", a little plastic portable bidet-type device, to keep the area clean.

"I had five stitches," says C, these, from an episiotomy. "It was fine. Most painful thing was the piles operation, five months later." Piles (haemorrhoids, lumps inside and around the bottom) after vaginal birth are, it turns out, very common; they develop because of changes in blood flow during the delivery, and because of the pressure exerted while pushing.

Once the head is out, the rest of the baby should be born relatively easily, the NHS thinks, usually within one or two contractions. Once the baby is all out: the NHS advises prompt skin-to-skin contact (holding the baby's flesh against yours, to regulate its temperature, breathing and heart rate, and to boost your oxytocin levels), and breastfeeding within an hour.

Oxytocin enables the breast milk to start flowing – this is the let-down reflex – in addition to which, hormone specialist Dr Nicky Keay tells me, it helps contract your uterus back to its normal size after you've given birth, which means you're not at risk of haemorrhage. "I remember," Dr Keay says, "the first time I breastfed, and I thought: 'This is quite cute! This warm little squidgy thing! Depending on me! I quite like this.' Then: I felt it! *I actually felt my uterus contracting!*"

"I'm speaking now as a woman who has birthed, and not from my midwife perspective, and I found the birth of my second daughter Aisha really healing," says the midwife Anna Kent (whose first daughter, you'll remember from the last chapter, died of a brain tumour when Kent was six months pregnant with her; Kent gave birth to her, she lived for an hour). "Afterwards, I felt triumphant. I birthed Aisha in hospital, in a pool, I had low-lighting, twinkly fairy lights, my [now] ex-husband wasn't there (his choice), which turned out to be positive for me; because I knew he would have been distressed by me vocalising pain. I think I would have opted for painkillers to appease him.

I was with a midwife friend who I knew and trusted, and I had a female birthing partner. I was mooing like a cow. I'm quite a calm person normally, I thought I'd be meditatively saying: 'Ooh, here's my baby!' The reality for me was screaming 'MY F*CK-ING FANNY!' And where else in life can you confidently scream that? I found it so liberating. And the women I was with were going: 'You're doing amazing, Anna!' And I was like: 'FOR F*CK'S SAKE!' And that was my positive birth experience. Anyone looking in could think, this is someone's Satanic ritual. Ha. But my experience of it was beautiful and no amount of pooing, or stitches, for me, could change that. I knew we were safe."

STAGE 3: AFTERBIRTH, WHEN THE PLACENTA COMES OUT

The third stage of labour is the bit in which the placenta – the organ that develops in pregnancy and provides oxygen and nutrients to the developing baby through the umbilical cord linking them – comes out, which, various mates tell me, not enough people ever talk about. I'd certainly never heard about it and S, mother of Cone Head the Baby-Barian, tells me she'd had zero idea it would happen, before it happened to her.

"So that was a shock."

The placenta comes out through contractions and pushing, just as the baby did. This is a process the NHS manages one of two ways: "actively" or "physiologically". "Actively" means you are treated medically, which makes it happen faster, with an injection of oxytocin into your thigh; "physiologically" means it happens naturally, and your body expels the placenta on its own.

Current evidence, the NHS informs me, suggests you shouldn't cut the umbilical cord immediately in the case of active management; medical professionals should wait between one and five minutes after birth to cut it and separate your baby definitively from the placenta (which had been keeping it alive, but which is no longer required). "This may be done sooner," it continues, "if there are concerns about you or your baby – for example, if the cord is wound tightly around your baby's neck."

The placenta itself will then detach naturally from the wall of your uterus, and your midwife will pull it out of you, through your vagina, using the umbilical cord. "Active management," it concludes, "speeds up the delivery of the placenta and lowers your risk of having heavy bleeding after the birth (postpartum haemorrhage), but it increases the chance of you feeling and being sick. It can also make afterpains (contraction-like pains after birth) worse."

In physiological management, where no oxytocin is injected, and everything is allowed to happen naturally, your umbilical cord will be cut once it has stopped pulsing, because that indicates it's no longer passing blood to your baby. This generally takes between two and four minutes. When your placenta has detached, you'll experience it as pressure in your bum, and you'll need to push it out, as you did your baby. This can take anything from a few minutes to an hour. If your placenta doesn't come away naturally, or if you start bleeding heavily, your midwife or doctor will advise you to switch to active management.

"The [oxytocin] injection is important to mention," Dr Wright tells me, "because increasingly people are choosing to have a natural third stage, physiological third stage. I always try and persuade people to [have the injection]. It speeds up the placenta coming out, but more importantly, it reduces the chance of you bleeding afterwards. Because if the womb's not contracting down, you've got that huge surface that's used to pumping out blood to the baby [still pumping out blood]. That's the biggest cause of maternal death worldwide. Apart from maybe (illegal, unsafe, unregulated) abortion – if we knew those statistics, but we don't."

STAGE 4: RECOVERY

This covers the first few hours after delivery. This is the skin-to-skin contact phase, the oxytocin phase, the point at which you may get stitches or other treatment for any tears or cuts in your perineum. "Your baby may have some of your blood on their skin and perhaps vernix, the greasy white substance that protects your baby's skin in the womb…" says the NHS website, "Mucus may need to be cleared out of your baby's nose and mouth."

CAESAREAN BIRTH

Those of you who have been paying attention will notice that what I, and the NHS, have been talking about to this point is vaginal birth, rather than caesarean. It was a caesarean that my friend R – whose contractions had been slowed by an epidural – ended up having.

"Twenty-four hours after the contractions began," she says, "the doc told me I would need a c-section. I was knackered and disappointed. A few hours later, I was whisked into the operating theatre with my partner, who was in scrubs. Needles went in everywhere, including (I assume) a sedative. The surgeon gave a full running commentary of what was happening; he explained to my husband which parts of my body he could see – 'And that's the bladder'. Swiftly followed by, 'This will feel like I am rummaging in a washing-up bowl'. There was a scrummage, then an almighty scream. The baby emerged. Still makes me well up when I think about it." And it was a caesarean birth that my friend P would have, after noticing greenish staining – meconium – in her waters.

Dr Alison Wright and Dr Shazia Malik tell me how they manage what they're trying to call "caesarean births" now, rather than "c-sections".

So what exactly does it involve?

"Caesarean birth is where we do a small cut, [along the] bikini line [on the mother's lower belly] and deliver the baby through that. Caesarean birth rates are rising around the world. Some of that's appropriate. I don't think anyone's really got the right to judge whether it is or isn't," Dr Alison Wright tells me. According to a 2021 WHO report,[42] "Worldwide caesarean section rates have risen from around 7% in 1990 to 21% today, and are projected to continue increasing over this current decade."

Anna Kent thinks "nationally we're looking at around a 40% caesarean rate right now, maybe higher," which, when I think back to those stories I collected from my friends' experiences, scans about right.

Why the increase? Are more women requesting caesarean births? I ask Dr Wright.

"Partly. We know much more about managing growth-restricted babies, and what the precursors to stillbirth are: reduced

---

42   Caesarean section rates continue to rise, amid growing inequalities in access, World Health Organization, 2021 – https://www.who.int/news/item/16-06-2021-caesarean-section-rates-continue-to-rise-amid-growing-inequalities-in-access

movements, for example. So we're intervening more to prevent those. It's for both reasons. Because women are requesting them, because we're doing them more – and also because we know they are much safer [than they once were]. Twenty, thirty years ago – the anaesthetic was not as safe, for example, whereas now, it's really safe. Just a spinal epidural. It's very safe in the UK."

So caesareans begin with an epidural. "Anaesthetists are brilliant at that – they test it."

How? "With ice [applied to the area, to check for sensitivity]. If it isn't completely, 100% effective, we've still got general anaesthetic as a back-up."

Can you give a woman in labour a general?

"It's not ideal. Pregnant women have more risk of aspiration." Aspiration is when something enters the lungs and causes an obstruction to breathing.

Because they carry additional weight? I ask Dr Wright.

"Because of weight; because of laxity of the muscles; because the larynx behaves differently."

Which was why pregnant women were particularly at risk during Covid?

"Exactly."

So, for the majority, a regional anaesthesia is given first, before the caesarean. What happens? Is there a screen?

"Yes, there," she says, motioning to indicate a small temporary medical screen positioned halfway down a body. "They can't see, anyway. We try and make it as natural as possible, which most people prefer. We try and drop the screen when we bring the baby out, some people like to try and push the baby out...

it means a lot to some people, to have that experience [of pushing]."

"When I do a caesarean," says Dr Shazia Malik, "I try and... this sounds slightly odd, but I try and do it like a normal birth. A lot of people talk about a 'gentle caesarean', but then, you watch the videos and... I don't think it looks that gentle. To me, a gentle caesarean is, you deliver your baby's head, and then it's very much like a vaginal birth – the less you do, the better. Because the female body is designed to do it! So you deliver the baby's head and then let the uterus and the baby do their thing."

Which is, to push? Because even if it's not a vaginal birth, the uterus is still contracting, still expelling the baby?

"*Exactly*," says Dr Malik. "The uterus is contracting, the baby is starting to wriggle, a lot of them will cry just when their head is delivered, or their shoulders are delivered. You get those shoulders out, and let the uterus squeeze, and the baby wriggle. It's beautiful, it's much better for the baby's chest, it's a much gentler entry into the world than doing it rapidly. It's tempting to quickly deliver the baby, isn't it? But actually, there's no need if we're not worried about the baby's health. If the baby's distressed and its heart rate is in its boots, you're not going to be doing this. The baby clearly needs to be out quickly. But, if you're doing a caesarean for reasons that are not going to affect how long it takes the baby to get out of the womb, it's much nicer to take your time."

How long? All in all? A couple of minutes?

"Yes! We do delayed cord clamping with a planned caesarean, routinely, if the baby is fine." That's waiting a bit, before cutting the cord, as the NHS site recommends with vaginal births. "But because it takes me two or three minutes to take the baby out, you've already done [the delay], often the cord will have stopped pulsating because we've let it do its thing."

Both Dr Shazia Malik and Dr Alison Wright tell me there is still stigma and misinformation clinging around the whole issue of caesarean births, even as the rates of caesareans increase (or maybe, precisely because they're increasing?). Both my friends C and M are mothers of two children, all born by caesarean. In both cases, their first were born by emergency caesarean, and their second, by elective (an unsurprising and direct consequence of the original emergencies), and I'd been *stunned* to hear how much opposition they'd encountered when expressing a desire to deliver by caesarean for the second birth.

"A midwife told me I wouldn't bond with my baby after a c-section," M tells me. "I had to have two counselling sessions before I could get it."

"They pushed me towards a natural birth at home," says C. "I was over 40. I'd ended up having one emergency c-section already. It seemed like madness. 'VBAC'. It's all f*cking 'VBAC!'"

What the living *hell* is 'VBAC'? I ask.

"Vaginal Birth After Caesarean," they say together, eyebrows raised, expressions dour.

So is there any legit reasoning behind all this? Ish. But really, truly, only ish. Regarding the less-good bonding theory, for example, there is, Dr Wright tells me, evidence fewer mothers breastfeed immediately following a caesarean birth. "From my understanding of it, it's because if you go through a long labour and then have a caesarean, you're more likely to be exhausted, or the baby might be – depending on the reason you had to have an emergency caesarean – the baby might have a problem, therefore you don't breastfeed. I don't think it's the caesarean itself." Overall, Dr Wright thinks, when weighing up the merits of caesarean versus vaginal births: "Everyone should be [more] aware of the effect of [vaginal] childbirth on long-term health. Some women end up pushing for a very, very long time, and we do know that can have a serious impact on the pelvic floor. If you're pushing for four or five hours, it's going to weaken your pelvic floor much more than if you're just pushing for an hour. It's often people's instinct to think: 'How's the baby? What's happening to the baby?' And if the baby's OK, 'We'll just carry on, push and push and push'. We don't care enough, in my opinion, about women's bodies, what happens to them in labour, what the long-term health implications of that are. Historically, we had targets [intended to limit the number of caesareans performed]. Until very recently, you had to have a certain caesarean section rate. Now, we don't, because we realised some poor junior doctor would think: 'Oh God, I'm not hitting the targets!' Then not do a caesarean, when it's really necessary. Those targets have all gone. WHO removed them."

In 2023, WHO released a statement saying that while, since 1985, "the international healthcare community has considered the ideal rate for caesarean sections to be between 10% and 15%...", it now believes, "every effort should be made to provide caesarean sections to women in need, rather than striving to achieve a specific rate... The effects of caesarean section rates on other outcomes, such as maternal and perinatal morbidity, paediatric outcomes, and psychological or social well-being, are still unclear. More research is needed to understand the health effects of caesarean section on immediate and future outcomes."[43]

The WHO ruling came in the wake of the UK's Shropshire Maternity scandal, a five-year investigation culminating in a 2022 report, which found that "mothers were denied caesarean sections and forced to suffer traumatic births due to an alleged preoccupation with hitting 'normal' birth targets."

The demolishing of targets sounds like a good thing, I tell Dr Wright.

"Yes! But people don't always realise it. And it suits some agendas to still have caesarean targets."

Whose? I ask – but she won't say, she is discreet and she is diplomatic.

"Ahem… midwives?'" suggest M and C. (I had not, I confess, realised quite how much tension can exist between gynaecologists, obstetricians and midwives, before I started talking childbirth with assorted interested parties. It is, one of them tells me, off the record, quite the toxic culture war.)

"If you look at social media, Instagram for example…" says Dr Malik, "there are some great people out there. But there's also a load of information out there that makes women think they've failed if they chose to have a planned caesarean section, they've failed if somehow their body didn't do what they thought it should do when they were giving birth… They'll go to classes and read stuff which tells them: 'Your body is designed to give you a perfect pregnancy and a perfect birth!' If your body always followed that design, if that were true, we wouldn't need midwives and obstetricians. The human body is not infallible, for

---

43 WHO Statement on Caesarean Section Rates, World Health Organization, 2023 – https://iris.who.int/bitstream/handle/10665/161442/WHO_RHR_15.02_eng.pdf

lots and lots of different reasons – none of which are your fault. None. If we look at caesarean section rates, they've gone up over the years. But there's always going to be a background caesarean section rate. And that's highest in your first birth, and that's because your body's never given birth before, so we don't know what it's going to do on the day. We don't know what your baby's going to do on the day. And we don't know what the two together are going to do on the day. I spend a lot of time talking to my clients about having an open mind."

Interestingly, exactly as rates of caesarean births rise, so a general, cultural preoccupation with "naturalness" in pregnancy and childbirth gains traction. The peak of this is embodied by the "freebirth" movement, the trend towards having your baby outside of the Western medical framework, entirely unmedicated, and without the intervention of a trained medical professional.

Why is this happening?

"Maybe it's come from over-intervention in the past… I think people have [moved on] from: 'I'm a doctor I know best'. I think some of my predecessors were quite arrogant. But I think now people want to do their own thing. It worries me that some women and people want to freebirth, completely away from any midwifery or obstetric support. Childbirth is a really risky business, potentially," says Dr Wright.

"If a woman wants to birth by herself in the woods, with the deer, she can," says Anna Kent. "If you want to birth at home with a midwife, you can (assuming a home birth service is available). If you want to birth in a hospital with all that modern medicine can offer, you can. People can birth however they want, and our role is to ensure informed consent, not to tell people what to do. I would support women and birthing people in whatever birth they chose. Freebirthing is where people choose to birth with no medical professionals in attendance, absolutely that is their choice to make. But it worries me if that choice is being made out of distrust for the medical world, as I feel that should drive us to make a better service so people *want* to opt in. I have seen births around the world (in refugee camps and conflict zones) where there is limited or no access to healthcare, and worldwide the biggest cause of maternal death is catastrophic bleeding after birth (also called PPH, postpartum haemorrhage). Sometimes a PPH cannot be predicted, and what concerns me about an unassisted birth is that the skill set midwives and other professionals have to stem the bleed may not be available."

At the same time, Kent says: "We have to acknowledge we don't always get it right in hospitals." How so? "The main naturally occurring hormone in birthing is oxytocin." Right. It controls contractions, the closing down of the uterus after birth, and kickstarts the production of breast milk. The whole shebang is dependent on it. "Yes. But stress – our fight or flight response – can inhibit the action of oxytocin, potentially an evolutionary thing so we can seek a safe place to birth. So…

"if the hospital environment is stressful, and the woman releases stress hormones such as adrenaline, this could potentially hinder her labour. Therefore, we know you're more likely to have a positive birthing experience, a safer birth, if you're in a low-stress environment…

"But in hospital that can be a challenge; bright lights, vaginal exams, someone talking about 'risks'… So here's the challenge; how do we create an environment where people feel empowered, listened to, and feel safe, but also where there is the medical input that may be required for birth?

"We know that dark lighting often helps so you don't feel exposed," Kent continues, "but sometimes medical professionals also need bright lights to see safely. Labour is driven by hormones, so the very act of our medical interventions may have a negative impact, that's why it is so important any intervention is offered on a case-by-case basis, and not a one-size-fits-all."

Yikes.

Not gonna lie, I say, ultimately. It all sounds a bit… completely horrific?

"Oh, it is," says one of my friends who's given birth.

As in: fully traumatic? I suggest.

"Pretty much," says another.

Why, then, did any of you go on to do it *again*, I ask, of those who did.

"Wanted more kids," says T, she of the pre-eclampsia, she whose husband was told he might have to choose between her and their unborn baby. "When they put J in my arms, I felt this ecstatic feeling washing over me; I remember thinking: 'Oh God, this is why I'm here!' I had a pretty vile family, mum and siblings. Suddenly, I thought: 'Now I can fill another one with love.'"

"There's such joy in seeing it – in seeing what the female body can do! I can't tell you!" says Dr Shazia Malik.

"It's beautiful. It really is," says Dr Alison Wright.

Not much arguing with that.

WHAT I KNOW NOW

- There are four stages of labour: established labour, delivery, afterbirth and recovery.

- The latent stage of labour is a warm-up act; established labour, Stage 1, begins when your cervix has dilated by 4cm. You'll know you've reached that stage because your contractions will be happening every five minutes (or more frequently), or your waters will have broken, or both. At this point, you should contact your midwife or maternity unit.

- Equally, if your contractions are further apart but very strong and painful, to a point where you need pain relief, or you're worried about anything, you should contact your midwife or maternity unit.

- Epidurals – powerful pain-relieving injections that go directly into the spine – can be given through earlier stages of labour, though not if you're getting close to the point of delivery.

- At 10cm, your cervix is considered fully dilated – enough for your baby's head to pass from your uterus into your vagina. Getting there can take 8–18 hours with a first baby; subsequent births tend to speed up.

- The second stage of labour is delivery of the baby. This is the point where you push. This generally takes around three hours for a first baby, two for subsequent babies – though this varies a lot.

- Women often say they're worried about pooing during this stage. Around 30% of them do, and midwives see this as a positive sign that the labour is progressing well.

- An epidural may mean that you don't feel that urge to push, in which case, medics may opt for an assisted vaginal birth – helping things along with a ventouse (a vacuum cup) or forceps.

- If your baby is delivered by ventouse, their head may be a little cone-shaped directly afterwards. This is called "caput succedaneum" or "scalp oedema" and generally settles down within days.

- When your baby's head is about to emerge, your midwife will tell you to stop pushing and instead take some short breaths, which you expel out through your mouth. This is to reduce the chance of your perineum, the skin between your vagina and your bottom, tearing.

- Massaging the perineum with oil before labour can help prevent this, too.

- Your midwife or doctor may ultimately need to cut this area, to prevent tears. This is called an episiotomy. You'll have a local anaesthetic for it, and stitches once the baby is born.

- Once the head is out, the rest of the baby should be born relatively easily, within one or two contractions. The NHS advises prompt skin-to-skin contact (holding the baby's flesh against yours, to regulate its temperature, breathing and heart rate, and to boost your oxytocin levels), and breastfeeding within an hour.

- Your boosted oxytocin will help your uterus contract back to its normal size.

- Stage 3 of labour is when the placenta emerges. This may happen physiologically, which means it comes out naturally, through contractions; or with some active medical intervention, i.e. a shot of oxytocin in your thigh to speed things up. An "active" delivery, is quicker and therefore, according to current medical recommendations, a safer option.

- Stage 4 of labour is recovery, and it refers to the first few hours after delivery. This is the point at which you may get stitches or other treatment for any tears or cuts in your perineum.

- Caesarean births currently account for around 30–40% of all UK births.

- They involve making a small cut along the mother's bikini line, her lower belly, through which to deliver her baby.

- They are generally performed after an epidural – a general anaesthetic in rare instances. They take around two minutes.

- There are no longer any targets regarding limiting numbers of caesarean births in the UK.

CHAPTER NINE

PERIMENOPAUSE AND MENOPAUSE

In the six years preceding the writing of this book, the conversation around menopause and perimenopause – the health stage all women hit, which marks the winding down of our reproductive lives – exploded.

It transitioned, if you will, from a shame-laden whisper, to a rowdy, raucous, solution- and medication-demanding din. From virtually nothing, to a furious outpouring over a long list of symptoms: hot flushes and hot flashes (What's the difference? I ask a doctor. "Flashes is American," she thinks), mood swings, interrupted sleep and itchy skin, brain fog, depression, anxiety, weight gain, the invisibility of menopausal women and the necessity (or otherwise) of "menopause leave" from work. We're now hearing a lot more about HRT, hormone replacement therapy, the most commonly prescribed medication for menopausal symptoms, and the alternatives to it (I have a mate currently microdosing magic mushrooms to treat hers). Then there's the spiralling industry around menopause, the endless, often overpriced products, the sheets designed to cool you down should you tend towards night sweats, the shampoos and skincare designed to specifically treat menopausal scalps, the vitamins claiming to offer "support" through what is now routinely referred to as "your menopause journey" – like it's a voyage of discovery, an X Factor entrant's back story, or a hormonal gap year, though it lasts a lot longer than a year. According to The British Menopause Society, symptoms of perimenopause and menopause typically last about eight years.

If the de-stigmatising of menopause is welcome, overdue, and desperately necessary – the unleashing of a barrage of intel, the clamorous noise, the rush to consider then re consider it, can also feel overwhelming. Add to this the fact that some women, some communities, are being totally left behind by it ("Who's talking to Black and Asian women about the menopause?" Dr Shazia Malik asked me); and… it's just a lot, isn't it?

Currently, I've got friends claiming to feel "very peri RN" the day after consuming a great deal of white wine (Me: "So is 'peri-menopause' what we're calling hangovers now?"). And I've got friends reduced to sleep-deprived, anxiety-addled shells by it; even one who has up to three migraines a week on account of it. I have friends in their early 40s driven crazy by skin – on their bodies, on their *faces* – which had started itching so horrendous-ly they wanted to tear it off with their own fingernails, and who had to beg for blood tests, because their GPs dismissed them as too young to be perimenopausal. I've got friends in their 50s who are completely untouched by it, and one who swears the undesirable symptoms are a conspiracy theory. "My periods have stopped – but who wanted them anyway?" she says.

And I've got friends – well, not so much "friends", as celebrity interview subjects – who knew literally nothing about it. In June 2024, I met Penny Lancaster, special police constable, broadcast-er and wife of pop star Rod Stewart; a woman who'd been so unprepared for menopause – which hit her like a truck, aged 49, in 2020 – she'd concluded that she was going mad. "I found that, one night after another, I was waking up, sweating from head to toe," she told me. "It wasn't just a little discomfort in the night. I was on top of the covers, feeling like this inferno was rising, as if I was standing in a pit of fire… I had a few… what I could classify as 'mental breakdowns'. We got chickens at that time and I remember hanging a hammock in the chicken area. I was the crazy chicken woman. If the kids wanted to know where I was, they'd find me wrapped up in this hammock, with the chickens. I couldn't cope with anything. Every time I woke up – the build-up of anxiety and fear! I've never been like that. I've always been like, 'It's OK!' People will come to me and say, 'I've got this sticky situation and I don't know what to do. There's this problem, Penny, solve it.' But I didn't have answers for myself, let alone anyone else." After being diagnosed as menopausal by her co-hosts on the TV panel show *Loose Women*, Lancaster sought help (and HRT), got her life back on track, and now campaigns for greater understanding of menopause, and access to treatment.

But – what actually is menopause? Why does it happen and why does it make some of us feel so sh*t, in so many different ways? I ask my experts.

"It's when your ovaries retire. They're not producing oestrogen and progesterone anymore," says Dr Nicky Keay. "It will present challenges."

"If puberty is the transition in life from childhood to physical adulthood," says Dr Charlotte Gribbin, "…going from being unable to reproduce, to being able to reproduce physically;

menopause is the opposite transition. You're going in the other direction, from being able to reproduce, to being unable to."

Right and: what's actually happening? Like, *inside*?

"We're running out of eggs," Dr Gribbin says.

"The loss of eggs with ageing – and the decline in ovulation – is the root cause of menopause," writes Dr Mary Claire Haver, author of *The New Menopause*. "This leads to hormonal shifts that impact every system in the body."

Because women are born with that finite number of eggs – and because that number starts dropping even before we're born (those eggs are already with us in the womb, making them technically nine months older than we are) – the decline continues through childhood, puberty and adulthood. By our early 40s, the 1 – 2 million eggs we were born with is looking more like 5000. At that point, the parts of our brain charged with rallying them, getting them impregnated and then secured within our uteruses every month, will be having an increasingly difficult time doing so. Eventually, they'll give up entirely, at which point, our periods stop.

On average, in the UK, women hit menopause at 51, but we could have been in the state of "perimenopause" for up to 10 years before reaching full blown menopause. During that decade, we may well have experienced some, or many, of those symptoms associated with it. It's also the case that menopause can start earlier than 51; menopause at 46 is considered to be within the range of normal by the medical community (menopause between 40 and 45 is called "early", and before 40, "premature"). Given the 10-year potential timespan on perimenopause, it's entirely possible to experience the symptoms of perimenopause from your late, maybe even mid, 30s.

"It's a pre-programmed point," Dr Gribbin continues, "where our brain starts to wind things down. We start to see changes in, guess what? Follicle-stimulating hormone, FSH, and luteinising hormone, LH. The bosses of oestrogen and progesterone." As they become less active, she tells me, our oestrogen slowly starts to come down.

Because it's just not needed anymore?

"Right."

"My way of talking about perimenopause," says Dr Sarah McKay, neuroscientist, "is this: we've got a constant conversation going on between the brain and the ovaries. And when you don't release an egg – because the ovaries have run out – a little trickle of oestrogen goes up to the brain, and the brain says: 'Release more!' And the signal goes back down to the ovaries, almost like: 'I can't hear you!' Then the ovaries go: 'OK!' and they release heaps. And the brain goes: 'Not that much!' And the ovaries go: 'OK!' Then the brain goes: 'No! More!'" This, she says, results in the rollercoaster of perimenopause, these "enormous fluctuations of oestrogen." Because our body is accustomed to a regular waxing and waning in oestrogen and progesterone over the course of a menstrual cycle – the one it's been dancing to since puberty – dwindling supplies of oestrogen, particularly, will cause it to have a freak-out… a multi-layered freak-out of many different expressions, which varies in severity, from woman to woman.

"Roughly speaking," Tom Bradley tells me, "25% of women will suffer badly from the symptoms of menopause, 25% will feel very little indeed, and the 50% in between will be on a sliding scale from mild to severe."

There are dozens – some say, *hundreds* – of symptoms of peri-menopause and menopause, and they accompany a change in the regularity, frequency and nature of your periods, which will ultimately end altogether (meno-stop, surely?). The NHS lists the more frequently observed symptoms – many of which I mention above – as:

- hot flushes, when you have sudden feelings of hot or cold in your face, neck and chest, which can make you dizzy

- difficulty sleeping, which may be a result of night sweats and make you feel tired and irritable during the day

- palpitations, when your heartbeats suddenly become more noticeable

- headaches and migraines that are worse than usual

- muscle aches and joint pains

- changed body shape and weight gain

- skin changes, including dry and itchy skin

- reduced sex drive

- vaginal dryness and pain, itching or discomfort during sex

- recurrent urinary tract infections (UTIs)

- sensitive teeth, painful gums or other mouth problems.

The NHS also mentions psychological changes, including low mood, anxiety, mood swings and low self-esteem, as well as "brain fog" – problems in focussing, concentrating and remembering.

It is – both Dr Nicky Keay and Dr Charlotte Gribbin agree – the dwindling of oestrogen that is responsible for all of the above problems. Oestrogen, you'll recall, is the good time party girl hormone, Maisie Hill's "Beyoncé of hormones". Its diminishment will not be lightly felt.

First, hot flushes, which are perhaps the most instantly recognisable and common among symptoms. They're the ones about which off-colour jokes are made, because they're dramatic and disruptive. "Top of the list," says Dr Keay.

Why does lowering oestrogen cause them?

According to Dr Keay, one theory is that your FSH and LH levels rise dramatically because they're trying to chivvy your ovaries into action. "The conductor of the endocrine orchestra, the pituitary gland, gets very cross with the ovaries: 'You're slacking! What are you doing?'" As a result, FSH and LH levels increase. And because the pituitary and hypothalamus act as the body's thermostat, constantly checking and adjusting its temperature, the theory goes that the brain's efforts to get the ovaries producing eggs – something they can no longer do – raises the body's temperature.

"Yes," says Dr Paula Briggs, obstetrician, gynaecologist, expert in sexual and reproductive health and – when I speak to her, in the summer of 2023 – chair of the British Menopause Society. "It's about the hypothalamus and thermoregulation. That's why they happen."

"Whyever they happen, the point is," Dr Keay goes on, "you feel out of control and horrible, typically in the middle of a meeting. And they disturb your sleep."

That loss of sleep will then be a contributing factor in a lot of the other symptoms. "Brain fog. Forgetfulness," says Dr Keay.

Low mood? I ask.

"It doesn't help. Oestrogen and progesterone are very import-ant for cognitive function and mood."

Progesterone, like oestrogen, falters in perimenopause and menopause: "a bit more erratically than oestrogen," Dr Gribbin tells me. Given the ferocious hold their influence has over our mood during the menstrual cycle – how incredible and confi-dent they make us feel at some points, how low and worthless, at others – it's not a complete surprise that their gradual, eternal, draining away from our system can have a significant impact on our mood, and – unlike menstrual cycle-related fluctuations in our sense of ourselves – these don't pass within a matter of days. They hang around, get entrenched, and start corrupting our confidence like fast-acting rot on a previously solid tooth.

Then there's:

"Headaches…" Dr Keay continues. I think of my mate and her migraines, how she has them more often than she doesn't, how she – a mother of two youngish kids – has to keep going regard-less. There is, sadly, little understanding of why women in meno-pause (and girls going through puberty, and women at specific points in the menstrual cycle) become especially prone to migraines; in the same way there isn't much understanding of migraines themselves. Fluctuations in oestrogen and progester-one are the most commonly cited cause; along with observations that migraines do seem to settle again, within two to three years after a final period.

And let's not forget: "urinary symptoms, needing to go to the loo more often," says Dr Keay. Because of a weakening pelvic floor? I ask. "Yes, but also because urinary systems are very close to reproductive systems," and changes in one can impact the other.

Then, she says, there's "vaginal dryness", an issue I last encountered when interviewing Dr Shazia Malik, who told me she'd experienced significant backlash after raising the issue of painful, post-menopausal, sex on a radio show broadcast in the Middle East.

Vaginal dryness – and the painful sex associated with it – happens in menopause and perimenopause because yet another one of oestrogen's extensive To-Do list points is the manufacturing of collagen, the great lubricator of your body. It keeps the mucosa – the tissue that makes up your vaginal wall – thick, elastic and lubed up; a lack of it will make that mucosa thinner, drier and more inflamed, which can result in painful sex, bleeding after sex; or just general discomfort – even when you're *not* having sex. This is what was once called "vaginal atrophy", but is now called GSM, the genitourinary syndrome of menopause; as referenced in Chapter 4.

Then, there's weight gain, and…

OH MY GOD.

Is this getting horribly depressing?

It is a bit, isn't it?

I'm sorry.

I'm going to get this crap over with, but hang on in there, will you, because then? I am going to get on to all the things you can do to help yourself, and there is A LOT. *So much*. As Dr Keay tells me: "The menopause is not evil." And for anyone thinking it all sounds like doom and gloom, Dr Keay reassures me that it doesn't have to be. "It's not an illness, it's not a disease."

"People are terrified of menopause," adds Dr Paula Briggs.

"They think they're going to lose their job and husband. That without HRT, their bones will crumble and their minds will go to mush. It's just not true."

> "Women win Nobel Prizes after menopause," points out Dr Philippa Kaye. "Go on to rule the world. This idea everyone's going to slide into dementia the moment they get menopause is not true."

I'm coming to this. No – really! I am. I *promise*.

But for now: weight gain.

"Oestrogen is pretty important for metabolism," Dr Keay tells me. So: because we lose oestrogen, our metabolism, our body's capacity to burn calories effectively, falters, and we gain weight? "It slows down – *and* we get more insulin resistance as our oestrogen goes down." Insulin resistance is when your body becomes less responsive to insulin, which can result in elevated blood sugar levels, because insulin's main purpose is to shift glucose from the bloodstream into the body's cells, where it can be turned into energy. If our body is resisting insulin, that glucose is going to be changed into fat, rather than energy.

"But also," Dr Keay continues, "if you're feeling a bit down and miserable, a bit 'I wish I could be 21 again', you're less likely to be motivated to exercise. So it becomes a vicious circle. And then you think: 'It doesn't make any difference if I don't eat this slice of bread – might as well eat the whole loaf.'" According to a 2022 study by ZOE,[44] post-menopausal women tend to have

---

44 Menopause and your gut microbiome: What happens?, ZOE, 2025 – https://zoe. com/learn/gut-microbiome-menopause-changes#

reduced diversity in their gut microbiome overall, but an increased level of certain bacteria – specifically *Dorea*, *Prevotella*, and *Sutterella* – all of which have been associated with obesity.

Then, there's the impact of stress on menopause, which is two-fold, according to an increasing body of academic study. A constant release of the stress hormone cortisol through earlier life can disrupt the production of oestrogen and progesterone – this is why stress can cause interruptions in a regular menstrual cycle and ultimately be a factor in preventing a woman from conceiving.

It now seems excess cortisol might also hasten the onset of menopause by up to four years. The second way in which stress impacts menopause is that we're more sensitive to it. Falling oestrogen can cause anxiety, which can make you more vulnerable to stress.

Then, there's the compounding factor of alcohol, towards which many women are inevitably, understandably drawn in perimenopause and menopause because: how else to deal with ALL OF THIS? However, the process of menopause makes us less capable of metabolising alcohol, because any associated increase in body fat means alcohol toxins are held in our bodies for longer, exposing us, for longer.

But IT'S OK! No, Really. Because there are other ways to deal with ALL THIS STUFF. Very powerful and effective ways.

"The first thing," says Dr Keay, "recommended by the British Menopause Society and the NHS – is lifestyle. Revise and review your lifestyle."

Diet. Exercise. Sleep. Stress management. The big four. The recurring theme on supporting the female body under any and all circs and life stages.

"Exercise can help hot flushes," says Dr Keay.

"Oh – exercise helps *everything*, all hormone disorders," Dr Briggs adds.

This is as good a time as any, I think, to note that pretty much every expert I have spoken to in the course of this work has, at some point or another, told me how vital exercise is to the good maintenance of a female body. I know this as a female body owner who herself started exercising at 40, and who has spent the last decade getting deeper and deeper into fitness, and more and more excited by how it can heal a person, physically and emotionally. Even when you pick up an injury – which I have – you can work around it and with it and through it, and end up stronger than you were before, so I'm going to say:

Women! PLEASE: *exercise*. Exercising is as important and non-negotiable as not smoking.

In terms of exercise, during perimenopause and menopause, Dr Keay particularly recommends: "Strength training, strength work." By this, she means weight or resistance training, any form of exercise that focusses on building physical strength. Lifting actual weights – dumb bells, kettle bells, bar bells, medicine balls – but also, using resistance to increase the effort you exert, e.g.: resistance bands, those massive rubber band-looking things, which you can tie around your thighs, then press against when you squat. I know all this stuff looks like Man's Business, intimidating and HOO-WAH! and grunty and *male*, but it is so important we start seeing it as ours too, our right, our duty to our bodies. Why? Because muscle mass in women naturally begins to decline when we are 30 (I know, I know), after which point, we lose between three and five per cent of muscle mass per decade. At 50, this accelerates to between five and 10%. This muscle loss engenders weight gain, as muscle is hungry – the more you have of it, in proportion to your body fat, the more calories you will burn. When that reducing muscle is combined with a reduction in bone density – yet another of the myriad gifts lowering oestrogen bestows upon the female body – *babe*. You're looking at an increased risk of mortality.

Back to Tom Bradley, physiotherapist, for his observations on how perimenopause and menopause impact the female musculo-skeletal system, and why strength training becomes so essential.

"Broad strokes," says Bradley, "what I'm seeing is, women in their early to mid-40s, coming in, and they're still having regular periods, but they've started picking up niggly injuries from things they don't understand... They're beginning to feel sore. They're beginning to pick up back and tendon pain. Tendon pain is something that's more and more common in perimenopause."

This, the medical community thinks, is because of how oestrogen starts faltering in perimenopause. The reduction in oestrogen comes with a change in muscle diameter. This, Bradley tells me, happens to men too. "If you took a 40-year-old man, and a 40-year-old woman, and you gave them the exact same exercise programme and monitored them monthly, both would get less cross section area of their muscles." But relatively, the drop would be greater for the woman.

In addition to which, bone density begins to drop in

perimenopause. Bone density is a measure of the amount of minerals, calcium and phosphorous, contained in your bones. Bone, when studied under a microscope, has a kind of honeycomb structure to it. The less healthy, and less "dense" it is, the bigger the holes in the honeycomb, and the weaker and more breakable the bone; this is also known as osteoporosis.

"Every woman has a different perimenopause and menopause, just like every woman has a different menstrual cycle," says Bradley. "But generally, bone density will start to reduce because you don't have the same amount of hormone, so aren't producing the same amounts of minerals."

I ask him what, then, we must do to help and: guess what he says?

You got it!

"Exercise. You need to maintain that muscular bulk by exercising, and you need to increase your bone density by weight lifting."

Because muscular bulk creates a barrier to injury, and weight lifting increases the density of our bones?

"That's it."

By the age of 80, 50% of women will have osteoporosis. Sorry but: Fifty. *F*cking*. Per cent. Oh, and wanna know what else? Should we, as older women, fracture a hip – far more likely, because of that escalating frailty in our bones – half of us will die within five years of that fracture. The survival rates for hip fractures in older women are lower than the survival rates of older women with cancer.

I started weight training in my mid-40s, not because I realised it was crucial to the healthy ageing of my skeleton, but because

I picked up a disc injury (while shaving my bloody legs – super common, Tom Bradley tells me). Part of my rehab training was deadlifting, the weight training in which you squat down and lift up quite a lot of weight – 20 kilos in my case – and I just... liked it. So I kept it up. But women, I think, are culturally squeamish about weight training. We're partly intimidated by it, and partly fearful that it will make us bulk up in a way that is socially unappealing. It is, in fact, *incredibly* hard to bulk up as a woman. You have to eat extremely consciously, consuming an enormous amount of protein, and lift extremely powerfully to achieve that kind of muscle. But, as one especially magnificent trainer says to me: "Hey, if you're *really* lucky and *really* devoted, you might just get there!"

But also? If it's a choice between bulging biceps, broad shoulders and osteoporosis? BRING ME THOSE KETTLE BELLS – right now. NO! THE HEAVIER ONES!

Where were we?

Ah yes.

The irony of perimenopause is that the one thing you need to do – exercise – is the last thing you feel like doing. Tom Bradley explains this is because you start picking up those niggly injuries, and sleep can be disrupted. Many of the changes that come with perimenopause, like shifts in sleep cycles and body temperature, make you feel off. It's similar to the luteal phase of the menstrual cycle, where your body temperature rises as progesterone fluctuates, but in perimenopause, this happens in slow motion. From a physiotherapy perspective, if you've got less muscle mass, weaker bones and your sleep is rubbish: you're more likely to get injured. So again, the one thing you *really* need to do, even if you don't feel like it, is exercise.

If this is the case in perimenopause – can I presume it only gets worse in full blown menopause?

"Yes. What I see in clinic is, you're not going to have the energy to do the amount of work required to compensate for your lack of hormone, which is making your muscles less strong and your bones less dense." This means: "People's bodies begin to change on them. And they start flogging themselves, or starving themselves, at the exact moment when actually, they need to be moving into a different form of exercise. They need to come up with an entirely new structure for it, to adjust their expectations of what their bodies can do. It doesn't mean that you can't lift – you *have* to lift. It doesn't mean that you can't run track, or do triathlons, or box… You *have* to. But you have to adjust your macrocycles. Your micro cycles."

Your "macrocycles" are the longish-term view on how you are exercising, eating, sleeping and recovering. So, Bradley recommends you look for patterns within that, evaluating everything you do in, say, a three-month period. You should record how many times you exercise, and what the nature of that exercise is, how it works in conjunction with other forms of exercise; and if you get injured, how long it takes you to recover. And: were you sleeping badly, or well; were you especially stressed? Were you getting headaches? Had you gone on a crash diet? (Lots of women panic about weight gain in menopause and go on extreme diets, but these often have the opposite effect. As Dr Keay tells me, "it scares your body, increases cortisol, and guess what that does? It's the 'let's save lots of fat, because this is an emergency situation' hormone.")

A micro cycle is the analysis of the same things over a shorter period of time – a week, typically. What Bradley is suggesting is a greater understanding of how various lifestyle factors affect your body in perimenopause and menopause. Keeping up exercise is key, but mixing in low impact activities – Pilates, yoga – with more intense workouts or weights will allow us time to recover. We can learn not to ask too much of a body that did not sleep well the night before, or the week before – but push it harder if it does feel rested and strong. Work out how and why you recover best, in this changed and changing body you now inhabit. On which note:

> "Sleep tracking is absolutely the most important component of recovery, bar none," Bradley tells me. So: "Sleep well, monitor your mood, monitor the general achiness in the body. And eat protein!"

Protein is essential in feeding muscle mass, it helps rebuild muscle after exercise whether you're male or female, menopausal or not; but in the case of menopause, it has the added benefit of helping your body produce hormones. NB: You don't lose all your hormones in menopause. "Oestrogen doesn't drop to zero," Dr Paula Briggs tells me. "You still produce some. Your testosterone *really* doesn't." It makes sense, therefore, to embrace a lifestyle which supports the hormones that are left.

"So, yeah: eat protein – and f*cking *talk* to someone!" Tom Bradley continues. "Because maybe you need HRT."

Ah, so: HRT. Hormone replacement therapy. The medical response to menopause symptoms. It's become so tightly intertwined with the discussion around menopause itself, it's like it's the same thing.

What is it?

"It's Ronseal," says Dr Philippa Kaye, GP. "Does what it says on the tin."

It's a Therapy that Replaces the Hormones lost in perimenopause and menopause?

"Yes."

So there's oestrogen?

"Always. Always oestrogen," Dr Kaye continues. "Oestrogen's the bit that makes you feel better, because it's generally what's causing the symptoms. Oestrogen has lots of roles in the brain. It tells you that you're not on fire, which mitigates hot flushes, and it has roles in libido, and all kinds of things. We have receptors for oestrogen from the hairs on our head to the skin on our toes. When we lose it, when our levels go lower: we know about it."

In the UK, all forms of HRT can only be prescribed by a doctor. Oestrogen will come either in the form of a gel, applied to the upper arm or upper thigh; or pills, taken orally; patches, which are generally applied to the thigh or bum; or spray, applied to the inner forearm. Which form you end up with will depend on your doctor's advice and, to a greater or lesser degree, what suits you.

"So everyone [on HRT] gets oestrogen," says Dr Kaye. "If you have a womb, you get progesterone," which tends to come in the form of oral tablets or in a combined patch with oestrogen and is sometimes also given (off licence) as a pessary into the vagina.

Why progesterone if you've got a womb? I ask her.

"Imagine: a lawn, that's the lining of my womb. It is grass seed [and oestrogen is like] light and water. So the lawn will grow and grow and grow [with oestrogen]. If I let the lining of my womb grow and grow and grow – I'm going to get some weeds in it. Oestrogen alone increases your risk of womb cancer. Progesterone is your lawnmower; it stabilises the lawn, the lining of your womb."

Gotcha. It is for this reason that women who have had hysterectomies – had their wombs surgically removed – will generally only be prescribed oestrogen.

What about testosterone? I ask. I understand some, but not all, women take it as HRT.

"At the moment, the guidance is that it should only be given for what's called 'hypoactive sexual desire disorder', which is: low libido. Testosterone has other roles in females, for example around muscle mass and metabolic rate. All kinds of things. Anecdotally, it seems that some women who take it report better energy, and less fatigue. They've got more va-va-voom. But for the moment, there is not enough evidence to suggest that it should be used for…"

The treatment of low va-va-voom?

"Ha. No, only for low libido."

When I spoke to Penny Lancaster, she told me that she was on testosterone, as prescribed by a private doctor, and that she was campaigning hard to get it more routinely prescribed on the NHS, too. Equally, I speak to a couple of other medically qualified individuals who aren't quite so convinced of testosterone's benefits. One of them told me she'd tried it, but it had made her really cross – so she knocked it on the head and only continued with the oestrogen and progesterone.

Your doctor – having diagnosed you either via a description of your symptoms or a blood test – will probably start you off with a lower dose of HRT, monitor how you respond, and adjust your dose accordingly. A major indicator of whether or not it is working will be, if any hot flushes subside – although this can take two or three months to become evident.

Like many medications it also comes with potential side effects, the most common of which are: headaches (which should subside within a few days), breast tenderness and pain, nausea (which should also subside within a few days), mood changes, muscle cramps, diarrhoea, mild rashes or itchy skin, and vaginal bleeding or spotting. Any concerns, go straight to your doc. Repeated and/or heavy unscheduled bleeding that persists after three months of starting HRT, go straight to your GP, as a matter of some urgency. Heavy unscheduled bleeding can be a consequence of the HRT, BUT it can also be due to things like endometrial or ovarian cancer, which need to be ruled out by a doctor.

On the subject of which, I say to Dr Philippa Kaye, and this comes from a place of profound ignorance, BUT: isn't there some broader association between HRT and cancer?

"Right. So. If you've had a hormone-responsive cancer like breast cancer, we generally say no [to prescribing HRT]. There are lots of non-hormonal prescribable medications for perimenopausal and menopausal symptoms, which can be recommended in the first instance. If you have tried everything, nothing's worked and you are still struggling, there is a conversation to be had with your doctor – for many women quality of life is most important of all."

Beyond that – it's OK?

"Every choice you make is a balance of risk versus benefit and you need to go through this with your doctor and come to your own decision, though I feel like HRT is a bit demonised."

Is that because society secretly doesn't want women to feel better, I ask; it just thinks we deserve to feel rubbish as punishment for not being able to have babies any more?

"Oh, no! That's too sad! No. I don't think that. I think that: a bad news story sticks. And it's got this generational memory to it. Like MMR," the measles, mumps and rubella vaccine, which was (completely, entirely, erroneously) linked to autism in a 1998 study by Andrew Wakefield, a study which was subsequently discredited, while Wakefield himself was eventually struck off. But that sort of thing, those sorts of stories: "feed into a mistrust of doctors and scientists. It sticks. Women who are mothers now, who may not have even been alive around the MMR issue – it's still something they know about."

Another one of those bad news stories surrounds HRT.

HRT has been around since the 40s; it's first form was a derivative of horse pee (really) called Premarin.

Adverts for it maintained it was a "cure" for menopause, that it could help a woman who felt "that her charm is gone, and the golden days of her womanhood are irrevocably past". With Premarin? "Breasts and genital organs will not shrivel. She will be much more pleasant to live with and will not become dull and unattractive." Hooray!

That early form of HRT was oestrogen only which – as Dr Kaye points out – was bad news in terms of increased risks of uterine cancers. This became clear in the mid-70s, after which point, progesterone therapies were introduced to balance the oestrogen. By the 90s, Premarin was one of the most prescribed drugs in the US. Evidence began to emerge that suggested HRT might help in the prevention of osteoporosis and also, heart disease; this lead, in the mid-90s, to the inception of a massive study, one which would become ground zero on this inaccurate but enduring narrative, linking HRT to an increased risk of serious, even fatal, illnesses.

The Women's Health Initiative trial was vast, the largest study of HRT ever conducted. It considered the impact of HRT on over 160,000 women aged between 50 and 79, over what was to be a course of 15 years. However, in 2002, researchers announced they were abandoning the study after only five years, because, researchers said, they'd observed an increased incidence of heart disease and breast cancer in women taking combined HRT – progesterone and oestrogen. These findings were widely reported in the press, vast quantities of women – understandably, terrified – stopped taking HRT instantly, throwing the medicine away, and doctors became incredibly nervous of prescribing it. It would subsequently transpire that the study's conclusions were massively flawed; the main issue being, the study was weighted towards subjects who were older than 60, meaning that women in their 50s, who tended to be healthier, but with more severe menopausal symptoms, were underrepresented. This meant that overall risks were exaggerated, and the risk/benefit balance (women with fewer menopausal symptoms, because they're over 60, and with less good baseline health, also because they're over 60, are not going to experience HRT as positively, as those in their 50s). The endocrinologist Megan Ogilvie would call the study: "One of the worst things to happen to women's health in a long time. It did a whole generation of women, and probably two generations of women, a huge disservice."

Also: "When you talk about oral HRT given to women in

their 60s," says Dr Kaye, "10 years after they've had any oestrogen, it's very different to giving it to women in their 40s and 50s whose bodies are still used to it. When you suddenly give oestrogen to someone who hasn't had it for a while..."

It's going to be a shock to the system?

"Right."

When it comes to womb cancer, Dr Kaye is clear: "as long as I give you progesterone: you don't have the same [risk]." She goes on to explain that the risk of blood clots in the legs – which can travel to the lungs – is a possibility with oral oestrogen. (It's also a risk with the contraceptive pill.) That's why doctors often steer clear of prescribing oral HRT for women who smoke or have other risk factors. In those cases, using oestrogen through the skin – like a gel or spray – can be a much safer option.

Cardiovascular disease is another area where perceptions are shifting: "if you're giving it to someone within a decade of menopause, HRT is actually thought to be protective against that," Dr Kaye explains.

And that leaves us with the biggie – breast cancer. Dr Kaye is keen to put this in perspective: "I think in any conversation about medication, we're talking about risk versus benefit. Always. There are risks in pregnancy. There are risks in unwanted pregnancy. There are women who take the pill for endometriosis, PCOS, and acne, whatever... For them the benefits [of taking the contraceptive pill] far outweigh those risks. And when it comes to HRT, it's the same. People often forget the huge benefit of controlling your symptoms. You're able to work. You're able to have your relationship. Your kids don't hate you. You're able to function. If you take 1000 women between 50 and 59, 23 of them will develop breast cancer, full stop. If you drink more than two units of alcohol, five more cases. If you smoke, three more cases. If you have obesity, 24 more cases. If you take HRT: four. So – it's small. But it's there. Yes, that risk is there. But when you weight it up against potential benefits, for many women it's worth it."

At the same time, both Dr Paula Briggs and Dr Nicky Keay wonder if HRT might be being overprescribed, certainly: over relied upon. "This idea: 'HRT is *The Cure?*'" says Dr Keay. "Take a whacking dose of it, straight away, guzzle this down, and almost – ignore the nutrition and exercise? To me, that is unsatisfying from the woman's point of view, because you want to feel in control of stuff, right? I'm very pro HRT – I'm on it myself – but it's the stages you go through. Sort out your life-style, feel empowered, now: 'I want to add in the HRT…' and I always say, start at a very low dose. Basic principle. Start very low, it might be that you may have to increase it: but only after three months. I get emails: 'I've taken it for a few days, it's not having any effect!'"

"I think that as well," says Dr Briggs. "It's good women are getting the information [on menopause and HRT], but the infrastructure isn't there to cope with it." The consequences of our suddenly being flooded with intel, she says, are "Very polarising. Women either can't get HRT, or they're self-administering doses that are much too high… I see clients with very high levels of oestradiol in their blood stream – and they're wanting [even] more!" There is something, Dr Briggs thinks, about HRT specifically, which makes women think they can just adapt and increase their dose at will, without medical guidance. "My hair-dresser recently said to me: 'I took two sachets of gel yesterday'.

I said: 'WHY?' She said: 'Good point'."

Like Dr Keay, Dr Briggs is not remotely anti HRT, but she does think it's being mischaracterised as the answer – when it isn't, always. "It's been over simplified. We want to believe it, too. But expectations are being pitched at the wrong level. If your BMI is over 35 and you've got diabetes – you're not going to be transformed by HRT. If you're overweight, then sweating is not uncommon" – so in that case, HRT might not make much of a difference. She also cautions against over-medicalising menopause as the root of all midlife symptoms – especially when it comes to mental health. "If the idea that managing menopause with antidepressants is wrong, which it is, then the idea of managing depression with HRT is also wrong. There's this campaign: 'Think Menopause'. But I think we also need to Think Outside Menopause."

Dr Briggs thinks we certainly need to *not* give hard-earned cash to the rapidly evolving menopause-branded commercial market – products like shampoo, vitamins, or menopause supplements. "A woman came to me and said she'd spent sixty quid on 'menopause bullets'" a variety of food supplement. "I said: 'just eat proper food!'"

Zoe did a vast study into nutrition in menopause in 2024, the biggest of its kind,[45] but fundamentally: good nutrition is achieved the same way in perimenopause and menopause as it is at any other point in your life: fruit, vegetables, good fat, limited sugars, limited ultra-processed food, anything that will help boost the variety of microbiome in the gut, and with that

---

45 Diet may counteract menopause metabolism change, ZOE study shows, ZOE, 2024 – https://zoe.com/learn/menopause-metabolism-study

additional focus on protein. In addition to maintaining a decent weight, exercising and having good sleep/recovery protocols, Dr Briggs says hypnosis and CBT, cognitive behavioural therapy, can help with menopause symptom management – especially important information for those with a history of cancer, which prohibits their using HRT. "There are also some new neuroendocrine drugs for treating hot flushes," she tells me. "These are non-HRT, non-hormonal..." so potentially, appropriate for women with a history of oestrogen-dependent cancers. "SSRI and SNRI antidepressants, they work for hot flushes and things," Dr Philippa Kaye tells me. "Anti-seizure medicines like Gabapentin... There are options."

Though, of course, in this case, as with all prescription medications, they should only be taken under a doctor's guidance.

Do menopause symptoms change over time? I ask Dr Kaye.

"In my head, I divide them into shorter term and longer term. Flushes, sweats, joint pain, headaches, depression, anxiety, all of those, are perimenopause and immediate menopause. Those tend to improve over time, though for about a quarter of women, symptoms can persist for many years, the average being around seven. Then, there's the impact of not having oestrogen over a longer period of time. That can lead to the genitourinary syndrome of menopause. Which can happen straight away – but often happens a bit later. Sore, itchy, burning, painful vagina, painful sex, UTIs, prolapses. Genitourinary syndrome of menopause is something we need to talk about more widely. Because women are miserable. Sex hurts, so their libido falls, because: why would you want sex if sex hurts? The physical and psychological aspects of libido are so closely interlinked. Even if it starts with one, it goes to the other, straight away. And that can have an impact on relationships. UTIs..." urinary tract infections, infections of the bladder, kidneys, or the tubes which connect them, "are not only miserable, they make older people delirious. And they can fall, which may lead to a broken hip, or a loss of independence and function and other issues." What can we do for those symptoms? "Vaginal oestrogen," a form of HRT, oestrogen, applied directly within the vagina. "It's really clear that vaginal oestrogen is safe, and it's safe long term. Later and later, with regards to the effects of long-term conditions related to the menopause you're thinking about things like osteoporosis."

Research has – and continues to be – conducted into the possibility that HRT helps protect women's bones from osteoporosis, and also our brains, from dementia. At the time of publication, no definitive conclusion has yet been achieved: though results are encouraging enough to warrant yet more research.

Now, one of the questions that inspired me to write this book was why the hell the rate of Alzheimer's disease in women is nearly twice that of men. Could it really be a response to falling oestrogen rates?

I'd better ask a neuroscientist.

WHAT I KNOW NOW

- Menopause happens when our bodies run out of eggs, and stop producing the hormones required to support those eggs through conception and pregnancy.

- It can make us feel rubbish. There are hundreds of symptoms associated with it, from hot flushes to anxiety and brain fog.

- Perimenopause describes the years which precede menopause, when we experience hormonal upheavals and associated symptoms.

- Perimenopause can last up to 10 years; though, on average, the entire phase of perimenopause into menopause lasts around eight years.

- Hot flushes are probably associated with the hypothalamus in the brain, which is the bit which orders oestrogen about, but which is also involved with the body's thermoregulation.

- Weight gain is another common symptom of menopause. It is believed to be a result of increased insulin insensitivity and a fall in gut microbiome diversity. It's also linked to tiredness from sleep deprivation, and the negative impact of mood changes (which make women less inclined to exercise).

- Exercise is vitally important to women in perimenopause and menopause, especially resistance training and strength training, which boosts the density of bones otherwise weakened by hormonal changes.

- So is good nutrition – with a focus on protein, which helps build essential muscle mass – sleep, and stress management.

- HRT, hormone replacement therapy, can also provide incredibly powerful relief from symptoms, when used in conjunction with good diet, exercise, sleep and stress management.

- HRT is not generally appropriate for women with a history of hormone-related cancers, but doctors will be able to advise on alternative treatments.

CHAPTER TEN

HOW THE FEMALE
BODY AGES

Ageing gets a terrible rap – really quite shockingly bad, have you noticed? – yet to this point, I think it is *marvellous*. Age has given me *so much more* than it has taken away. I like how I look, I like how I feel – I *love* how I move around the world, knowing *it*, and knowing *me*, better and better all the time.

Liking us both, better and better, all the time.

If the hangovers are worse – the confidence is insane, solid and suffusing. If age is expensive – the optician's bills, the spiralling supplements, the subscriptions to wearable tech tracking my biometrics to keep me "optimal", and on, and on – it's also a liberation. Like Gwyneth Paltrow once said (ahem, to me) in an interview: "I don't give a f*ck. I don't care. I've turned 50, I don't give a fu*ck what anybody thinks."

Honestly? In my experience? Age isn't merely a privilege. It's a massive advantage, and it is a *trip*.

CANCER AND AGE

But, I am writing as a woman who hasn't yet encountered any major sickness in her life. As we age, our risk of developing conditions like cancer increases. In fact, age is the biggest risk factor for cancer, with over 90% of cases diagnosed in people aged 45 and above. Breast and skin cancers are those most likely to affect women; we addressed how to self-check breasts in chapter 5 – how boobs work – where we also covered the importance of attending routine mammograms. A side note on skin cancer: in 2024, the charity Cancer Research UK reported a significant increase in melanoma skin cancer diagnoses over the course of the past decade. The figure rose by 57% in the case of the over 80s, a statistic which CRUK attributed to that generation being the first to go on cheap package holidays, while knowing almost nothing about the dangers of sun exposure. Simultaneously, at the other end of the age spectrum, the 18–25 brigade have most unexpectedly and unwisely reinvigorated the dangerous trend for sunbed tanning. In 2024, a survey[46] commissioned by cancer charity Melanoma Focus revealed that, while 28% of UK adults use sunbeds, which sounds like *loads* to me... *43% of 18- to 25-year-olds use them.* Which is mind-blowing. There's even a TikTok trend called Tanning Thursday, which both urges young people to get onto a tanning bed in preparation for the weekend, and somehow collates the practice with ideas of wellness and selfcare. There is absolutely no mention of the fact that sunbeds were categorised as Group 1 carcinogens in 2009, or that people who start using sunbeds before the age of 35, have a 75% increased risk of developing malignant melanoma.

Women are more likely to get skin cancer than men, and much more likely to get breast cancer. Ninety-nine per cent of breast cancer cases are in women. We can also be subject to five forms

---

46 28% of UK adults are using sunbeds as skin cancer rates rise, Melanoma Focus, 2024 – https://melanomafocus.org/news-blog/28-of-uk-adults-are-using-sunbeds-as-skin-cancer-rates-rise/

of gynaecological cancer. The Eve Appeal – the UK charity devoted to gynaecological cancer – explains on its website that there are five types: womb cancer, ovarian cancer, cervical cancer, vulval cancer and vaginal cancer. It describes the most common symptoms of each like this:

Womb cancer
- Bleeding after the menopause, like blood in discharge (pink, brown, red)
- Bleeding between periods
- Bleeding that is unusually heavy for you
- Vaginal discharge that is blood-stained

Ovarian cancer
- Unexpected increased abdominal size and persistent bloating (not bloating that comes and goes)
- Feeling full quickly, loss of appetite or feeling sick
- Pelvic and/or abdominal pain
- Needing to wee (urinate) more often
- Changes in bowel habits

Cervical cancer
- Vaginal bleeding during or after sex – this is often the first sign
- Bleeding in-between periods
- Bleeding after the menopause, 12 months since your last period
- Lower back or pelvic pain

Vulval cancer
- A lasting vulval itch

- Pain or soreness
- Thickened, raised, red, lighter or darker patches on the skin of the vulva
- An open sore or growth visible on the skin
- A mole on the vulva that changes shape or colour
- A lump or swelling on the vulva
- Bleeding or blood-stained discharge inbetween periods or after the menopause (when you haven't had a period for 12 months or more)

Vaginal cancer
- Unexpected vaginal bleeding
- Vaginal discharge that smells or may be bloodstained
- Vaginal pain during sexual intercourse
- A vaginal lump or growth that you or your doctor can feel
- A vaginal itch that won't go away
- Pain when urinating (peeing)
- Persistent pelvic and vaginal pain

Should you have any of these symptoms, or more general symptoms, like fatigue or unintentional weight loss, you must, of course, go and see a doctor.

It should also be said, after that grisly list, that cancer disproportionately affects men.

Men have a one in two chance of being diagnosed with in their lifetime – while for women, the chances are one in three – and men are more likely to die of cancer than women. Both these discrepancies are thought to be a consequence of lifestyle.

Men are more likely to smoke, and smoke more, also to drink, and drink more, both smoking and drinking massively and negatively impact cancer rates. As for those mortality rates: men are less likely to see a doctor to discuss symptoms early on – at the point where cancer is more easily and effectively treated. By the time they do tip up for medical attention, this means any cancer is more likely to have spread. This is, of course, rubbish for men, and for those of us who find ourselves attached to one or two in particular, but it does also speak to the positive impact of being aware of your body, engaged enough to notice when it changes, and proactive enough to seek help when you need it. Also of not drinking much – or smoking, at all.

HEART DISEASE

I couldn't, however, write about women's cancers, without also writing about coronary heart disease. Coronary heart disease is the main cause of heart attack; and it is twice as likely to kill women, as breast cancer. It's also more likely to kill women than men. This is because women are more likely to delay seeking medical attention – possibly because they are less aware of how myocardial infarction presents in women, and how that differs from presentation in men – and they are 50% more likely than men to receive an initial misdiagnosis. Both men and women are 70% more likely to die following any initial misdiagnosis. According to research[47] from the British Heart Foundation, it is estimated that, over a 10-year period, more than 8,200 heart

---

47   Heart attack gender gap is costing women's lives, British Heart Foundation, 2019 – https://www.bhf.org.uk/what-we-do/news-from-the-bhf/news-archive/2019/september/heart-attack-gender-gap-is-costing-womens-lives

attack deaths in women across England and Wales could have been prevented had those female patients received an equivalent standard of care to men. "The study found women were less likely to receive standard treatments including bypass surgery and stents," reported the BHF. Women who smoke, have high blood pressure, and diabetes are at a considerably greater risk of developing heart disease than men with the same conditions, and...

No. It is not fair. Biology, apparently, is no great respecter of fairness. This info is, however, definitely worth knowing; it is also worth reacquainting yourself with Dr Charlotte Gribbin's description of myocardial infarction in women, in Chapter 2. It's also worth knowing that a defibrillator should be used on bare skin, and that if attempting to use one on a woman, you should (according to the St John Ambulance) first remove all her clothing, including her bra.

ALZHEIMER'S DISEASE

As mentioned earlier, part of the reason I started thinking about this book in the first place was because I saw a statistic claiming women are more likely than men to get dementia – the neurodegenerative disease associated with ageing, which causes a loss of cognitive abilities such as thinking, remembering and reasoning. Twice as likely, according to the UK's Alzheimer's Society. Out of pure selfishness – I really, *really* don't want to get dementia – I'd fixated on that figure. What explained it? Hormones, again? Brain structure? Social pressure, the rigours of pregnancy, childbirth and child raising, overloading our systems to the point of fusing, just pure impalpable womanliness... *WHAT*?

"Let's look at Alzheimer's disease in particular," says Dr Sarah McKay, neuroscientist. "Dementia is an umbrella term, used to describe lots of these diseases of ageing." Alzheimer's is a specific type of dementia, one characterised by a progressive loss of memory. It is a disease of the brain – that's why I'm asking a neuroscientist about it.

So: is it true that women get Alzheimer's more frequently than men?

"It's true that more women than men are diagnosed. Part of that is, women live longer than men. There are more old ladies alive to get dementia, than there are old men." According to the ONS, the Office of National Statistics, the life expectancy of women in the UK is between three to four years longer, on average, than that of men. This is generally explained in the same way as those cancer statistics, above: by women's tendency to be healthier, and pay more attention to their health, to be more engaged with medical services, to drink less, smoke less, and even eat better. (A 2024 study into gender differences in food preferences found that while men preferred red and processed meat, women preferred vegetables, whole grains, tofu, and high-cocoa-content dark chocolate, all of which are demonstrably healthier.)[48]

"So if we look at sheer numbers, there appears to be a propensity there."

What else? Might it be hormonal? Might it be that our brains and bodies, which are accustomed to being flooded with oestrogen in our youth, fade away when its levels decline after menopause? There are a lot of oestrogen receptors in our brains, right,

---

48   Assessing gender differences in food preferences and physical activity: a population-based survey, *Frontiers in Nutrition*, 2024 – https://doi.org/10.3389/fnut.2024.1348456

and if scientists are investigating whether HRT helps prevent Alzheimer's – is it connected to menopause? Activated by it?

"We only really started looking at brain scans of menopausal women about two years ago [in 2021]. We really lagged behind in asking [those] questions. Menopause [brain scans] came out of the lab of a woman called Lisa Mosconi."

Dr Mosconi is also a neuroscientist; she's published a lot of books, 2024's *The Menopause Brain*, among them. In 2021, she led a team of scientists that scanned the brains of 161 women aged between 40 and 65. The resulting research, Mosconi has said, observed "changes in structure, connectivity and energy production (which falls, but stabilises or even rebounds in later years for some). And the greatest brain changes occur in the timeframe where [menopause] symptoms are most intense." Dr Mosconi's research: "has shown that, for women with a predisposition to the disease (a family history or genetic markers), red flags for Alzheimer's start appearing in the brain during the menopause transition. Whether the same applies to women without a predisposition, we don't know, but are looking into it. Importantly, while all women go through menopause, they don't all develop Alzheimer's (about 20% do). So meno-pause does not *cause* Alzheimer's, but it may make the brain more vulnerable."

One of the things Dr Mosconi notes, was that grey matter becomes fatter again in perimenopause.

"Which is kind of really weird," Dr McKay tells me. "It's the reverse of puberty and pregnancy," when grey matter thins, allowing the brain to make faster connections and essentially sharpen up. The re-thickening of that grey matter makes those connections slower again, which naturally begs the question:

Do we get more stupid during menopause? I ask Dr McKay. "No. As your hormones are dialling down … we do see this grey matter bounce back" – but we also see the changes that happen during perimenopause, when menopause symptoms are at their most intense – "we also see that flatten out. The brain adjusts."

Dr McKay believes that what happens to our brains during and after menopause, including our risk of developing Alzheimer's, may be impacted by the amount of hormone to which we've been subject earlier in our lives.

"Things like the pill and hormones get a bad rap, but actually, oestrogen's a cognitive enhancer. So for women with high levels of oestrogen, on the pill or during pregnancy, we often see cognitive enhancement." (Dr McKay has already told me: "If you have a pregnancy, you'll get a thousand time more oestrogen than you'll receive in the entire rest of your life. And our brains *really* like oestrogen." This influx of oestrogen, specifically the subset oestradiol, is particularly evident in the third trimester of pregnancy, apparently.)

"At the end of the life, if you look back, the more doses of oestrogen you've had over the lifespan, you see resilience to ageing. It's neuroprotective."

Which can help protect your brain against diseases like Alzheimer's – and which is why there's some thought, hope and research, into whether HRT does the same.

Dr Mosconi says, "Taking HRT solely to prevent Alzheimer's disease is not currently recommended," but points to a study, published in 2023[49] by the organisation Frontiers in Ageing Neuroscience, as reason to at least continue researching the possibility. This study, a "Systematic review and meta-analysis of the effects of menopause hormone therapy on risk of Alzheimer's disease and dementia", concluded "Results of the present meta-analysis suggest that oestrogen therapy initiated during the critical window of the menopause transition may support neurological function and reduce the risk of future AD [Alzheimer's disease] among eligible women."

Dr McKay also wonders if Alzheimer's is more prevalent in women, because it's more routinely diagnosed in women – and because of the part we play in society. "There's a really interesting theory that a mate of mine called Kate Gregorevic has here in Australia." Dr Kate Gregorevic is a geriatrician and internal medicine physician. "She sees a lot of older people come to her office, people who've emigrated, and don't have English as a first language. And particularly the more traditionally structured families, if the female gets Alzheimer's disease, she often comes to the clinic much earlier in the disease process, than the man. Because if the man still has his wife getting up every morning, making him his tea and his toast, washing his clothes, he presents much later, because he's kind of supported through. Whereas if she gets dementia, he's screwed. So we see gender playing a role there in terms of diagnosis. But we can't say, 'Oh [you got it], because you've got two X chromosomes.'"

---

49 Systematic review and meta-analysis of the effects of menopause hormone therapy on risk of Alzheimer's disease and dementia, *Frontiers in Aging Neuroscience*, 2023 – https://doi.org/10.3389/fnagi.2023.1260427

She also thinks there's reason to be hopeful that Alzheimer's will become less apparent in women, as our societies become more equal in gender terms. "The gender gap is closing in terms of a lot of these diseases of ageing. You don't get to your 80s without having a history of life experiences – biological, social and intellectual – that got you there. We all carry these risk factors and these protective factors from our lives. You look at a woman who's 80 now: how many years of education did she have, compared with a man of the same age? Which country in the world did she live in? How many pregnancies did she have? How many children did she raise? Did she have a really intellectually stimulating job? How was her overall biological health, in comparison to a male? My generation: I'm nearly 50. Mine and my husband's experiences are far more similar now, than our grandfathers' and grandmothers' – even our parents' experience. What we see in men, is, they're starting to live a little bit longer. Women have always lived longer, but that gap is closing; because men are smoking less, they're drinking less, they're not working in mines." And as women have more interesting, educated, connected, out-in-the-world lives than we used to, lives more like the ones men have lived historically: we'll be less likely to develop Alzheimer's?

"Look at what the Queen did."

Dr McKay and I are talking in the year after Queen Elizabeth II died. She was 96, had ruled the UK for 70 years and 214 days, had met with her private secretary to discuss the imminent induction of new Prime Minister Liz Truss less than 48 hours before dying, and had apparently been working on State Papers in her bed until the very moment of her death, pretty much. "Men typically die like she did; live, then don't have a very long illness before they die. The Queen did it in 24 hours. She's the perfect example. Women typically aren't like the Queen. Often, there's a few more years of ill health in those extra years. You don't want that. You want your health span to match your lifespan. The Queen is the perfect example."

The Queen had other things going for her, brain-health wise, Dr McKay points out.

"She had four children. Up to four children builds in biological resilience to ageing – it makes your brain look slightly younger – but if you have more than four, the stress of it all wipes that. Though I suspect for someone like the Queen, even if she'd had six children, it wouldn't have been that stressful. Because she had so much help."

Beyond that:

"She was born into the right postcode, into wealth and privilege. Socio-economic status is one of the strongest indicators of health outcomes. She was incredibly engaged, she had the best healthcare anyone could have on the planet, she was physically active… She did all of the right things. Some of her own doing, some by virtue of who she was. And she worked up until the day before she died, and I would love to be like that."

Me too!

"Wouldn't that be the dream?"

But assuming we're not the Queen, and we haven't had four babies (no more, no less): what else can we do, to increase our brain health? To protect it against Alzheimer's, and everything else? "One, understand how much your expectations and experiences play into your perceptions of health. That's not to say that it's all in your head. But – to understand that often, you can't just say: 'Oh it's hormones', or 'it's this one aspect of biology'. Two, I don't think it matters at which point of lifespan you're at, often the strongest indicator of good health and a good experience of going through a stage of life, is social relationships."

Decent friendships = good brain health?

"Yes. During puberty and pregnancy, the parts of the brain that are changing, are the social brain. We have this absolute biological mandate to connect. It's not just a little baby who needs to be nurtured when it's born: a mother needs to be nurtured too. Nature doesn't want us to parent alone. The risk factor on PND" post-natal depression, "or teenage angst, is loneliness. Social isolation. We often look at, I don't know, some Silicone Valley dude bro type who wants to 'optimise every aspect of his physiology'... When if we looked at the social networks we build around us – they're actually the strongest indicators of good health. We need healthy warm relationships – they're the biggest risk factor and the biggest opportunities for great health."

This, apparently, is the reason hearing loss can be a prediction of dementia. It's not that the loss of hearing itself is connected with cognitive decline, it's that an individual with hearing loss can withdraw from social situations, become isolated, and lose those healthy warm relationships.

As well as a good social network – sustaining a sense of purpose is proven to provide a strong defence against cognitive decline.

A 2022 study published by researchers at University College London, which reviewed eight previously published papers, including data from 62,250 older adults, across three continents, found that a sense of purpose is associated with a 19% reduction in rate of clinically significant cognitive impairment. See the Queen for further details.

Anything else, I ask Dr Sarah McKay.

"Three: the other one is sleep. If you haven't, from a biological standpoint, got sleep sorted, everything else will be much harder to do. It's the foundation all brain health is built on. Sleep is the price we pay for brain plasticity: we go to sleep every night, our brains get kind of flushed out, cleansed out, when we are asleep. It's when our memories of the day get wired in. We all know how bad we feel if we miss one night of sleep: so you really need to focus in on that. If you can get the social and the sleep right, you're 80% of the way there."

In addition to everything we've already covered about muscle loss and osteoporosis, and how to support and manage them with exercise and nutrition, and post-menopausal hormone levels, and how to manage *them*, this amounts to desperately important intel on how best to approach ageing, on how to mitigate and manage its issues, on how to best protect our bodies and our brains from its onslaught.

WHAT I KNOW NOW

- Ageing is not nearly as bad as society would have you believe, actually: it's rather brilliant. (NB: I knew that before. Gwyneth Paltrow told me.)

- But age *is* the biggest risk for cancer. Nine in 10 cancer diagnoses are in people aged 45 and above.

- Skin cancer is on the rise, and disproportionately affects women, particularly those over 80. It's also becoming more common in younger women, possibly due to the fact that 43% of 18- to 25-year-olds use sunbeds, a major risk factor for skin cancer.

- Men are more likely to develop cancer than women, and more likely to die of it; but the five kinds of cancer which almost exclusively impact women are womb cancer, ovarian cancer, cervical cancer, vulval cancer, and vaginal cancer.

- Women are twice as likely to die of coronary heart disease than they are breast cancer.

- Women are also twice as likely to be diagnosed with Alzheimer's disease as men.

- There are ongoing studies into whether HRT helps protect the female brain from Alzheimer's. They are, as yet, inconclusive, but promising enough to merit further research.

- Neuroscientist Dr Sarah McKay believes that the narrowing gender gap between men and women, will result in fewer women being diagnosed with Alzheimer's.

- Sleep, and good, meaningful relationships, and a sense of purpose have all been shown to help protect the brain from Alzheimer's.

EPILOGUE

So – that's it, then?

Presenting the complete workings of the female body! Top to toe! Hormone to hormone! Puberty to old age; mood swing to ACL injury to mid-cycle oestradiol high to assisted vaginal birth! The whole shebang; the works, the lot!

Except that: it isn't. *Of course,* it isn't. Two years and a ton of interviews later, I know infinitely more about how the female body works than I did when I started… but I also know how much more there is yet to know. Some of which, *no one knows.* Though they're trying, they're really trying.

But what a ride so far, eh? What a wonderful thing the female body is. So intricate and funny and competent and clever and cool. Much more magical again, for not being magical at all. For being a meticulously calibrated machine, which changes and grows and can even grow whole other iterations of itself! Which messes up – then makes itself better, given half a chance. Fails, and reasserts itself. How beautiful, how glorious, how fragile, how tough.

* * *

When I introduced this book, I talked about my body being like a car I was driving around, with zero comprehension of how it did the things it did, and no desire to read the manual. Actually?

I'm not sure that was true. I think I didn't entirely trust that my body, any of our bodies, really could be understood. That there *was* a manual. I think I thought female bodies were unknowable and wilful, rogue and illogical. Ageing cantankerous bits of tech no one could ever get to work entirely right.

But I don't feel that anymore. I have glimpsed beneath the bonnet – and I understand so much of it! I know there is logic there! Individual, erudite and very involved, sometimes defiant, counterintuitive – but, nonetheless! LOGIC. There is so much about our bodies that *just makes sense.*

Like:

The hormonal ballet, the influence it wields over our life – our movements and our moods.

The differently shaped feet, which should not be squeezed into any shoe made without respect for their particular anatomical requirements.

A brain which changes format, over and over and over again, depending on its circumstances. A schedule, which must be adhered to, programmed deep into our DNA.

And while I still don't know why oxytocin is described as the "warm and fuzzy" hormone (is that literal? Are our nerve endings gently triggered by it, so they "fuzz"? Does the thermoregulation function of our hypothalamus respond to it by raising our body temperature a smidge?), or why childbirth hurts so much when it is so essential to the propagation of humanity (JUST MAKE IT EASIER AND WOMEN WOULD WANT TO DO IT MORE)… What I know above all, now, is this:

Knowing more about your body, better understanding it, how it does what it does, *why* it does what it does, can only make you respect it more. It can only make you admire it more. It can only make you want to do the right thing by it, more.

Support it. Feed it. Move it. Rest and relax it. Throw everything you've got at letting it do what it does, to the best of its ability. Heal it. Advocate for it. Take it out dancing! Take it for a long walk. Take it to the docs, if you're worried. Pop it in the bath if you're stressed. Love it, as much as you can. Be civil to it, at the very least.

ACKNOWLEDGEMENTS

With extraordinary gratitude to the experts who gave up their time, their extraordinary knowledge and their experience, to talk to me. Thank you, thank you:

Tom Bradley, Dr Paula Briggs, Dr Sharon Cox, Professor Hilary Critchley, Anna Deignan, Dr Charlotte Gribbin, Dr Catherine Hill, Maisie Hill, Professor Andrew Horne, Dr Kate Jolowicz, Megan Jones, Dr Philippa Kaye, Dr Nicky Keay, Anna Kent, Dr Shazia Malik, Professor Hilary Marland, Dr Sarah McKay, Sophia Money-Coutts, Dr Tara Porter, Professor Dame Lesley Regan, and Dr Alison Wright.

Also to:

Robert Lee, to whom, I took the contract.

Elisabeth Perlman, a tireless, phenomenal researcher.

New River books! Rebecca Nicolson and Aurea Carpenter, for getting in touch in the first place, then guiding and cheerleading me on; Helena Sutcliffe for exceptional editing. Katherine Stroud and Ella Chapman for top-notch marketing and promoting.

Tone, for always just letting me get on with it.

And Nicola Jeal (without whom, nothing ever really happens).

ABOUT THE AUTHOR

Polly Vernon has been a features writer, interviewer and columnist for 18 years. She now writes primarily for *The Times* and *Grazia*. She started as a junior writer on *Minx*, a riotous young woman's magazine, which launched in the late 90s as a female response to Loaded. Since being picked up as the *Guardian*'s youngest ever Comments and Analysis columnist, she has written for every publication from *Vogue* to *The Telegraph*, and has interviewed everyone from David Cameron to Katherine Ryan via Donald Trump.

INDEX